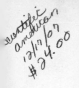

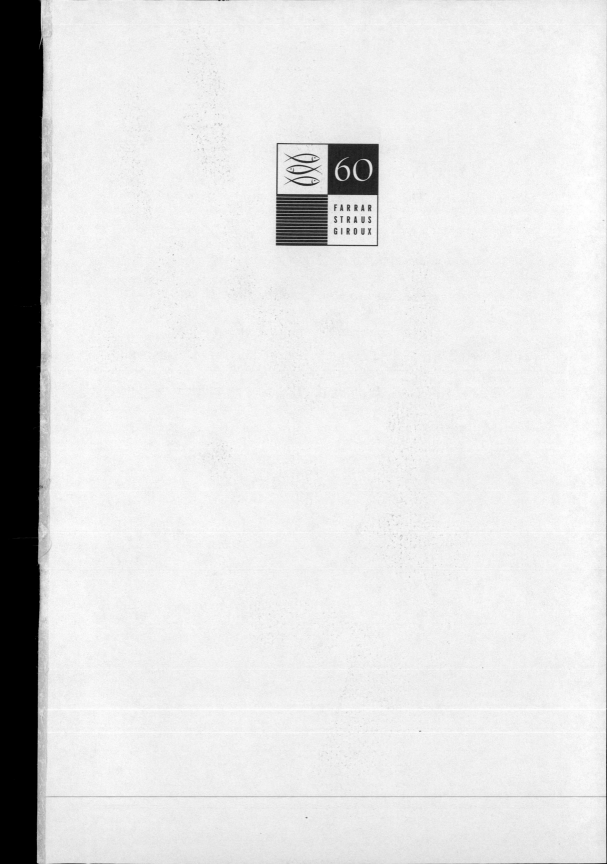

RETHINKING THIN

RETHINKING THIN

The New Science of Weight Loss—

and the Myths and Realities of Dieting

GINA KOLATA

Farrar, Straus and Giroux | New York

Farrar, Straus and Giroux
19 Union Square West, New York 10003

Copyright © 2007 by Gina Kolata
All rights reserved
Distributed in Canada by Douglas & McIntyre Ltd.
Printed in the United States of America
First edition, 2007

Library of Congress Cataloging-in-Publication Data
Kolata, Gina Bari, 1948–
    Rethinking thin : the new science of weight loss—and the myths and
realities of dieting / Gina Kolata. — 1st ed.
        p.   cm.
    Includes bibliographical references and index.
    ISBN-13: 978-0-374-10398-9 (hardcover : alk. paper)
    ISBN-10: 0-374-10398-4 (hardcover : alk. paper)
    1. Weight loss—Psychological aspects.   2. Reducing diets—Psychological
aspects.   3. Health behavior.   I. Title.

RM222.2.K576 2007
613.2'5—dc22

                                                          2006033816

Designed by Jonathan D. Lippincott

www.fsgbooks.com

1   3   5   7   9   10   8   6   4   2

To Bill, Therese, and Stefan

Contents

RETHINKING THIN

Prologue

Three obesity researchers were having breakfast at a medical meeting in Charleston, South Carolina, a few years ago when their talk inevitably turned to the Atkins diet. It had reached a new peak of popularity, and they were simply annoyed with the diet and the whole low-carb movement. It just irked them that this seemingly irrational way to lose weight, this seemingly unhealthy, if not dangerous, diet scheme, was being hailed as the secret to effortless and permanent weight loss. The whole Atkins movement was built on testimonials, they groused.

"We kept saying, 'Nobody has any data,'" said Gary D. Foster, who was the clinical director of the weight loss center at the University of Pennsylvania. Finally, the three decided, Why not do a study? They had not applied for funds, but they were curious enough to do some research anyway. "It would be quick and dirty," Foster remarked, just a brief look at whether the Atkins diet had any value. The three fully expected to discredit it, showing it was no better, maybe even worse, than traditional diets for weight loss, and dangerous to boot. They just knew that the diet was going to do something awful to cholesterol levels and that people who followed it were going to be risking a heart attack.

And, they slowly realized, they also would be asking a question that, amazingly enough, had never been asked in a rigorous way: Is one diet any better than another? You might think that with all the years, all the *decades*, of obesity research, the answer would be obvious. It's a question that, of course, would have been well studied. But you would be wrong. That question, that fundamental question, had just been left dangling.

And so it began, the first attempt to compare the Atkins diet with something more traditional, the standard low-calorie, low-fat diet beloved of academic weight loss clinics.

The study took place at three medical centers—the University of Pennsylvania, the University of Colorado, and Washington University in St. Louis—and was directed by the three doctors who conceived it. It was small, involving just sixty-three obese men and women, people whose average weight was 216 pounds. And it lasted for one year. The subjects were randomly assigned to follow the Atkins diet—the researchers handed them the book *Dr. Atkins' New Diet Revolution*— or to follow a diet and behavior modification plan written by Kelly Brownell, a Yale psychologist who publishes an earnest textbook-like manual called *The LEARN Program for Weight Management*. "We picked LEARN because it is the most frequently used manual [at weight loss centers]," Foster explained. "It is the gold standard for weight loss and behavioral weight control."

No one could have been more surprised than these researchers when they saw the results.

The Atkins diet, they discovered, seemed better than the usual diet program, at least for the first six months; the subjects' weight loss, an average of 7 percent of their body weight, was twice as good as with the low-calorie diet. Granted, no one lost much weight, and granted, 40 percent of each group dropped out, and granted, by the time a year was up, the two groups were about equal in their total weight loss and almost everyone in either group who lost weight had regained most of it. The Atkins dieters ended up, on average, losing 4.4 percent of their body weight, or about 9½ pounds, and the low-calorie dieters lost about 2.5 percent, or about 5½ pounds, but the difference between the groups was not statistically different. Still, the Atkins diet, to the investigators' astonishment, led to higher levels of HDL cholesterol, which is linked to protection against heart disease, and lower levels of triglycerides in the blood, which also indicate a reduced heart disease risk. The conventional diet did just the opposite.

"That's not what we expected," Foster said. "How did it happen? Was it good? Was it bad? Was it indifferent?" And, most important, "What *is* the best way to lose weight?"

This last one is a fraught question, of course. To someone like Gary Foster, tall with a long, gangly body and barely a hint of a paunch, a man who does not worry about his weight, the question is of academic interest. It is a research puzzle, a query that could lead to more grants for his university's weight loss center, which paid his salary, and that could lead to publications in leading medical journals, bolstering his professional reputation. But for the millions of overweight people who have spent their lives obsessing about food, veering from one diet, one weight loss plan, to another, thinking about food and their weight every day of their lives, the question is all too immediate.

The three researchers published their results in the May 22, 2003, issue of the *New England Journal of Medicine*, one of the most prestigious medical journals. Their paper was accompanied by an editorial that ended with the usual platitudes. "The recipe for effective weight loss is a combination of motivation, physical activity, and caloric restriction," it said. "Until further evidence is available regarding the long-term benefits of a low-carbohydrate approach, physicians should continue to recommend a healthy lifestyle that includes regular physical activity and a balanced diet."

The editorial, of course, dodged the question. Is it possible for most people to permanently lose weight? And, if so, how? If "a healthy lifestyle" were enough, would two-thirds of the nation have a weight problem? Would the nation be gripped by what is often called an obesity epidemic, as evidenced by the grim statistics of a growing national girth? The percentage of people who are overweight or obese was a whopping 47 percent in the period from 1976 to 1980, but now it is an even more whopping 64 percent.

The overweight say it is not that they don't try to be thin. All they do is try, many say, but nothing seems to help.

They may never have asked whether there is any scientific evidence that one diet is better than another, but most have, in a sense, experimented by themselves, trying diet after diet, hoping to find one that will lead them to their dream weight. They long for the weight that would let them buy clothes in the size they think is really them, or that would give them the sort of confidence in their weight loss that would let them enjoy an ice cream cone without the dread that just a taste of a forbidden treat will set off an out-of-control eating binge, or that would allow them to eat Thanksgiving dinner without the dismal conviction that they will pay for every bite with extra pounds.

They are like Linda Lee, a *New York Times* writer, who tried the Atkins diet. It worked, but then she backslid. "I just had to have a piece of bread, a slice of pizza, a muffin, and the weight came back." She went on "the punishing Ornish no-fat diet," but after losing weight she gained it back again. She bought prepared meals that were made according to the Zone Diet; she went to Weight Watchers. She even tried self-hypnosis, to no avail. The next plan? "I am going back on the Atkins diet."

The knotty problem was described in a report on obesity treatments by the National Academy of Sciences. Its committee of medical experts concluded that the battle for weight control is never won, even after you lose weight. "An obese individual faces a continuous lifelong struggle with no expectation that the struggle required will diminish with time. For most people, even a brief abatement in effort will be met with a significant setback in control."

Yet there are those who manage to rid themselves of extra fat, like Richard Wurtman, director of the Clinical Research Center at the Massachusetts Institute of Technology. Wurtman got control of his weight decades ago and has never regained the pounds he lost. He is by no means naturally thin; he says, "I am a fat man in a thin man's body." But, somehow, he beat what groups like the National Academy would describe as overwhelming odds. Was it he who beat the odds, or was it his methods?

So the three obesity researchers—Gary D. Foster, James O. Hill of the University of Colorado, and Samuel Klein of Washington University—decided to put the Atkins and low-calorie diets to the ultimate scientific test. They would do a larger study, this time enrolling several hundred obese subjects, enough so that the conclusions would not have to be hedged. They would not just hand people the diets to try on their own but would provide them with intensive counseling and support, an expensive and demanding program that is thought to give the best hope for sustained weight loss. The subjects would follow the Atkins diet or a low-calorie one, and the study would last two years, long enough to get some idea of how well any weight loss held up. Like the initial pilot study, this would be a randomized clinical trial, the most rigorous of clinical studies, in which the subjects would not choose their diets but would be randomly assigned to them.

This is the story of that clinical trial, some of the people who joined it, why they thought they were fat, whether they lost weight, and whether, in the end, one diet was any better than the other. But it is also the story of what came before and what is coming next. It is a story of the weight standards set by fashion and medicine, the lessons learned by science, and what all this means for dieters.

The saga of people's unending attempts to control their weight is a tale of science and society, of social mores and social sanctions, of politics and power. It raises questions of money and class, and of whether there is such a thing as free will when it comes to eating and body weight. It raises questions of how and why the discoveries of science, which have slowly chipped away at the reasons for obesity and the real health effects of being overweight, have been shunted aside by marketing and hucksterism and politics.

And it is a story of the secret world of the overweight, who fantasize about finally, at long last, getting thin. What is it like to know the calorie count of every morsel of food you see and to worry that a single spoonful of ice cream or a cube of Swiss cheese can send your eating spiraling out of control? What is it like to face, as the National Academy of Sciences so bluntly put it, a *"continuous lifelong struggle with no expectation that the struggle required will diminish with time"* (emphasis mine)? And how did our society, today, end up with what may be the greatest disconnect ever between the body weight ideals that are held up as obtainable if you really try and the body weight realities for most people?

This is a book about what it is like to be fat in this country today. It is about the nature of the current fixation with obesity, where it came from, and why it persists. It is about personal obsession and social obsession with body weight. And it is, in the end, about obesity— a scientific and social phenomenon that has defined our time, made some rich and others miserable, led to the elation of discovery and the despair of dashed hopes when easy answers did not arise. It is a story that begins with a research study and one newly hopeful dieter.

1

Looking for Diets in All the Wrong Places

If you met Carmen J. Pirollo, you might not realize that he has a weight problem. He's a square-jawed, animated man, who talks in exclamation points, favors preppy clothes, and—the big hint that he's a bit self-conscious—sometimes doesn't tuck in his shirts. Yet while you may notice his abdomen under that shirt, he is not what you might think of as obese. He does not seem to have any trouble moving, and when he sits down, he does not spill out of his chair. He's not like one of the subjects in those insulting, deliberately humiliating photos that show up in magazine articles or on television programs to illustrate the horrors of the obesity epidemic—those familiar images of round-faced, double-chinned people captured stuffing hamburgers into their mouths or of a fat family lumbering past fast food restaurants, dipping into bags of popcorn or licking ice cream cones.

But Carmen, according to the official standards, is fat—obese, in fact—and he knows it. He's 5 feet 11 inches tall, and at 265 pounds, his body mass index, a measure of body fat based on height and weight, is 37. That is a level at which public health guidelines warn that dire health risks start to mount.

And dieting has become a part of Carmen's life. Over the years, he has tried almost every variation on the dieting theme, losing weight over and over again, only to gain it all back, and more. "I've lost a whole person over my lifetime," he says. In his thirty-two years of professional life as an elementary school teacher at a New Jersey school not far from his townhouse in Philadelphia, he has seen his weight climb and climb and climb despite all his efforts to control it.

But on a chilly evening on the first day of March in 2004, Carmen, at age fifty-five, opened a new chapter in his weight loss history. He began a two-year stint as a volunteer in the extraordinary experiment that was prompted by the small pilot study a few years earlier comparing the Atkins diet with a standard low-calorie one.

The three investigators who did the first study got federal funding to expand it to include 360 obese subjects at their medical centers—the University of Pennsylvania, the University of Colorado, and Washington University in St. Louis—and continue it long enough to get some answers that would hold up to scientific scrutiny. They'll follow each subject for two years, with regular measurements of weight, blood pressure, kidney function, and stamina. They'll periodically question their subjects about satisfaction with the assigned diet, and they'll evaluate the dieters for changes in mood.

The two diet plans could not be more different. The low-calorie diet program is one that few dieters have heard of but that is beloved by academic researchers. It was developed by a member of the club, a university professor, not some self-promoting diet doctor, but a *researcher*, a psychologist whose goal was to give the best advice for weight loss, whether or not it was what fat people wanted to hear. And it comes with a hefty manual that tells you how to succeed, culling the accumulated wisdom of academic researchers. The diet's name is as earnest as its advice. LEARN, it's called, which is an acronym for "Lifestyle, Exercise, Attitudes, Relationships, Nutrition." And it was the diet with which Atkins would be compared.

Of course, no one signing up for the new study wanted the low-calorie LEARN diet. They were attracted by the idea of a two-year intensive program to help them lose weight and keep it off. They knew their diet, Atkins or low-calorie, would be decided at random. But they were hoping they would get Atkins, the diet that all America at that time, it seemed, was adopting. The Atkins diet was developed by a man so confident in his program that he called it "the new diet revolution."

The Atkins diet plan says that carbohydrates make you fat, so you must strictly limit them. But you can eat your fill of other foods.

You will be counting grams of carbohydrates, but how hard is that when you can fill up on foods like steak and eggs? Also, Atkins promises, you won't be hungry. No more going to bed at night feeling famished, hardly able to wait for the next morning when you can eat again. No more obsessing over the next meal, feeling a gnawing hunger even as you finish your meager allotted portions of the meal you are eating. His diet, Atkins stressed, was *nothing* like those food-deprivation diets that almost everyone who struggles with their weight has tried and tried again. His diet really was a program you can happily follow for the rest of your life. "With Atkins, you'll get the results you've dreamed of without the agony of deprivation," he insists.

LEARN's message is that if you want to lose weight, you have to face up to a punishing reality—you probably will never be eating your fill, and you will always be keeping track of what you are eating and how much. You will always feel that edge of hunger. But the program will teach you how to manage. You will learn to monitor your food, and to stop eating before you are sated. You will learn tricks, like putting your fork down between bites of food, that will slow you down and help you eat less. You will learn to recognize portion sizes: what a 4-ounce piece of steak looks like, or a medium apple, or a 1-ounce slice of bread. And that training will stand you in good stead for the rest of your life as you try to keep your eating under control. "Let's face it—losing weight is hard work and maintaining weight loss can be even more challenging," the LEARN manual bluntly says.

Atkins says that carbohydrates are diet traps, making you put on weight despite yourself. If you greatly reduce the amount of carbohydrates you eat, he promises, your body's metabolism will change so you start burning your own fat for energy and you lose weight.

LEARN says that the source of your calories is not the issue—it is how many you are eating that matters. Consuming too many calories is what makes you fat, and if you want to lose weight, you have to count them rigorously every day. There are no forbidden foods, but your goal is to eat healthfully, so you are to choose foods consistent with the U.S. Department of Agriculture's food pyramid while keeping careful track of your calories. That means keeping a food diary, weighing and measuring what you eat, and choosing foods that are low in fat. It means a diet that emphasizes fruits, vegetables, grains, and cereals.

The advice embodied in LEARN is pretty much what has been urged upon Americans for decades, yet it is advice that few have followed. STRIVE FOR 5 say the cheery signs in Wegmans food markets, a chain of supermarkets in the Northeast, exhorting customers to eat five or more servings of fruits and vegetables each day. But if you just turn your head, you will see the warm loaves of bread piled behind the bakery counter, the cheese breads and oil-coated focaccias next to the long loaves of French bread, which, as almost every dieter knows, are made without fat. And scattered about the aisle of apples— thin-skinned red McIntoshes, next to speckled Cameos, next to shiny green Granny Smiths, next to a pile of ovoid Pink Ladies—are little plastic pots of caramel dip. Life is hard for the resolute.

But the LEARN program was never supposed to be the academics' answer to fad diets that promise miracles. It began about as modestly as a diet can, as part of a Ph.D. dissertation by a young psychology student at Rutgers, New Jersey's state university. The year was 1976, and the student, Kelly Brownell, was testing the hypothesis that dieters would be more likely to succeed if their spouses got involved with their weight loss program. The idea was to help spouses be enablers, and not dissuaders, by teaching them to keep temptations out of the house, to prepare low-calorie foods, and to help the dieters eat three measured meals a day with only preplanned snacks in between.

So Brownell wrote a diet-and-behavior-modification program for all the dieters in his study to follow and a companion program for spouses. His plan was to recruit overweight people and, in keeping with the rigors of scientific research, assign them to different programs. One group would get the diet program and behavior modification program along with a companion program for their spouses. Another group would get the diet program and behavior modification, but their supportive spouses would have no special instructions or training. There also would be a third group of dieters, people who wanted to lose weight but whose spouses said they were completely uninterested in helping in any way. Those subjects would get the same diet and behavior modification as the others, but in all likelihood, they would get no additional help or support at home.

The program manual was all-important to the study because it was the key to making sure that everyone got the same weight loss advice, no matter who administered it. The three groups of subjects would meet with different facilitators, so Brownell had to be certain that they were told exactly the same things about diet and behavior modification.

"We basically wrote a protocol on how to deliver treatment for obesity," Brownell says.

The study got under way. Brownell recruited ten obese men and nineteen obese women, with an average age of forty-five and an average weight of 208 pounds. The weight loss treatment phase of the study lasted ten weeks, with weekly ninety-minute sessions on diet and behavior modification. That was followed by six months of a maintenance program, with monthly meetings.

As Brownell expected, people did best when their spouses were actively involved—that group lost, on average, 20 pounds in the first ten weeks and another 10 in the six months that followed, losing twice as much as the group whose spouses were not cooperative or those whose spouses were involved but were not taught how to help.

Brownell's dissertation went smoothly—he handed in his neatly typed Ph.D. thesis, he sailed through the requisite grilling by faculty members, and his study was published in 1978 in *Behaviour Research and Therapy*. He ended up with a faculty position at the University of Pennsylvania, where he continued his research on how to lose weight and maintain weight loss. But, to his surprise, the manual that he wrote for his dissertation was becoming a hit at academic medical centers.

"One of the most interesting outcomes was that people wanted this book on how to do behavioral therapy. We started to copy it and send it out, but we were breaking our bank just sending it out. We started asking people to pay for photocopying, and then we started revising it, making it longer because we were learning more. Soon we started to ask, Should this get published?"

But publishing the manual as a book was problematic, Brownell realized. What was the point—to have his book become part of the vast ocean of diet books that appear each year and then vanish, out of print? To have his book, if he was lucky, appear on a table of new books in bookstores, then move to the store's shelves, first displayed face out, then with just its spine showing, and then piled in a remainder bin? And were eager dieters really going to grab a book about a program called LEARN, a program that says that weight loss should be slow and steady and that maybe you will never get to the weight you think is your goal, but losing even a few pounds is good for your health?

"Diet books have a short half-life. You have to have a gimmick, and you have to do what Atkins did, find a diet that makes people lose weight really fast," Brownell says. (He says the Atkins gimmick is to place such stringent restrictions on what people can eat that they end up eating many fewer calories simply because so many of their favorite foods are off-limits.)

Yet academic researchers wanted the LEARN program, and Brownell wanted to provide it. He decided to form his own publishing company, American Health Publishing Company. By publishing the manual himself, he could keep his book in print, revise it every year, and make it, he says, "user friendly."

"We put all the expertise in there, but in an engaging, optimistic, even humorous format," Brownell says. There are cartoons—*Cathy* and *Garfield* are particular favorites. And scattered little boxes of text give helpful hints with headlines like "Did You Know?" ("Did You Know? Underestimating your daily caloric intake by as little as 100 calories a day can add more than 10 pounds of body weight each year.") It looks like a high school textbook, not a typical diet book, and there are no inspiring tales of dramatic weight loss or lives transformed by the diet. The chapters end with little quizzes, and dieters are given homework, like a form at the end of Chapter 2 in which to write down what they ate; what time they ate it; their "feelings"; their activity, if any, while eating; and the calorie count of each meal. They get a list of the calorie content of foods, and they get advice on sticking to the diet that is not particularly revolutionary but, Brownell says, has proven to be useful—keep tempting foods out of the house, shop when you are not hungry, keep records of what you are eating, get regular exercise.

Brownell also took pains to be strictly ethical about his program. As founder of the company, he explains, "evaluations by me would be a conflict of interest." But other academic groups evaluated the program, with results, Brownell said, that varied from place to place and context to context.

"Sometimes it was the main treatment. Sometimes it was used in the control group. Sometimes it was used with medications. Sometimes you get very skilled people using it, and sometimes you don't." So it remained on the scene, familiar to obesity researchers, unknown to most of the public, rarely criticized, generally accepted, and with an air of wholesome, earnest healthfulness. It was, of course, nothing like the story of the Atkins diet.

More than a decade before Brownell wrote his program, a New York cardiologist, Robert C. Atkins, was trying to lose weight. He read about a low-carbohydrate diet in the *Journal of the American Medical Association* and tried it on himself in 1963. It worked, he said— pounds just evaporated. So he decided to remake himself as an obesity doctor. He turned his medical practice into an obesity clinic, putting his own patients on the diet. Then he wrote a book promoting it. Published in 1972, *Dr. Atkins' Diet Revolution* told people they could eat all the fatty foods they wanted as long as they kept a tight rein on their carbohydrates. By keeping their carbohydrate levels down, Atkins said, people would keep their insulin levels down and would keep hunger at bay. The book was an immediate bestseller, and immediately raised the ire of academic medical experts, who said the diet was crazy and dangerous and that its high fat content would lead to high cholesterol levels, which in turn would cause heart attacks and strokes.

In 1973, the American Medical Association's Council on Foods and Nutrition published a blistering critique of the diet, calling it a "bizarre regimen," saying Atkins's ideas were "for the most part without scientific merit," and adding that while Atkins claimed that the diet would activate a fat-mobilizing hormone, removing fat from storage, no one had ever found such a hormone in human beings.

In April 1973, Atkins was called to testify before the Senate Select Committee on Nutrition and Human Needs. He appeared with his lawyer and said he stood by everything in his book, including his advice that pregnant women could safely go on the diet. Leading obesity and nutrition experts were appalled, testifying that Atkins's diet was dangerous and that they were aghast at the idea of telling pregnant women to follow it. "If I were a fetus, I would forbid my mother to go on such a diet," Karlis Adamsons, an obstetrician at Mount Sinai Medical Center in New York, told the Senate committee.

The diet's popularity waned after that, but then it waxed again. Atkins kept it before the public eye with his bestseller *Dr. Atkins' New Diet Revolution*, published in 1992 and again in 1999. Along the way, he founded a company, Atkins Nutritionals, to sell foods and supplements. But nothing about his program, his self-promotion, or his company sat well with academic medical experts, and his program retained a whiff of the unsavory, of quackery.

That began to change shortly before Atkins's death on April 8, 2003, after a fall resulting in a head injury. It was a time when everyone, it seemed, who had ever struggled with his or her weight was on a low-carbohydrate diet.

The low-carbohydrate fad began with a remarkable development, an article in *The New York Times Magazine* that seemed to vindicate the doctor and his diet. Written by Gary Taubes, a freelance writer who himself was on the Atkins diet, it was published on July 7, 2002, to immediate controversy in some circles and acclaim in others. The magazine's cover featured a juicy steak, glistening with fat and topped with a pat of melting butter. "What If It's All Been a Big Fat Lie?" the article was titled, and it argued that, in fact, fat does not make you fat. Carbohydrates are the culprit. The obesity epidemic was caused by the emphasis on low-fat diets, which, paradoxically, made people overeat.

Atkins was gleeful, proclaiming on his Web site that he had been proved right after all those years of derision:

Sunday, July 7, 2002, was one of the most gratifying days of my life—and one that validated the controlled carbohydrate nutritional approach to weight management and good health. This watershed article in a mainstream consumer publication accurately describes the scientific basis and effects of a controlled carbohydrate lifestyle, mirroring my conclusions from 40 years of clinical experience: The low-fat belief system causes individuals to over-consume high carbohydrate foods, which in turn has contributed to the current epidemics of both obesity and diabetes.

For months afterward, television shows, magazines, and other newspapers discussed the low-carbohydrate hypothesis, reciting dieters' reports that they had shed pounds nearly effortlessly when they gave up carbohydrates and dutifully noting nutritionists' excoriations, their fears that the diet was unhealthy, that it would promote heart disease, and that weight loss with this diet would never be sustained.

Meanwhile, the latest edition of Atkins's book, *Dr. Atkins' New Diet Revolution*, appeared in paperback and shot onto bestseller lists. It was, of course, nothing like the earnest LEARN manual.

In the Atkins books, the message is exuberance, enthusiasm, cheerleading. The books feature inspiring case histories of people Atkins says were typical dieters who followed his program. He says he gave them pseudonyms. He also provides no details to convince a skeptic that what the dieters said was true, or even that these patients really existed. But their stories helped drive home the message. This diet, Atkins was saying, really works.

So, in his *New Diet Revolution* he tells of "Tim Wallerdiene," who lost 122 pounds in nine months and kept the weight off for two and a half years. His cholesterol level went down, and so did his blood pressure. The back and neck pain that had plagued him was gone. "I'm a better dad and husband," he proclaims. "My old phrase used to be, 'No, I'm not up for that.' Now I love to play with my children."

Atkins makes exciting promises: "Lose weight! Increase energy! Feel great! This book will show you how it's done."

And he claims that the diet passed scientific muster. "Atkins works because, as an increasing body of scientific evidence shows, it corrects the basic factor that controls obesity and influences risk factors for certain diseases. That risk factor is insulin."

Then, in May 2003, the small pilot study comparing the Atkins diet with a low-calorie one appeared in the *New England Journal of Medicine*. For doubters, for those who worried that a low-carbohydrate diet might not be safe, that publication, in the nation's most prestigious medical journal, gave the diet a new legitimacy. It said that over the short term, at least, those who followed the diet did *not* end up with soaring cholesterol counts and they even seemed to lose *more* weight than the low-calorie group.

For the three researchers who conceived of the pilot study, those data inspired them to start their larger study. For millions of overweight Americans, the study inspired them to start a low-carbohydrate diet on their own.

By the time the Penn study began in 2004, low-carbohydrate diets were booming. Twenty-six million Americans claimed they were on one. At that time, when enthusiasm for the diets knew no bounds, sales of books promoting low-carbohydrate diets and specialty low-carbohydrate foods and beverages were expected to reach $30 billion. The low-carbohydrate dieters said they did not care if they were getting 40 percent of their calories as fat, nor did they care if the diets restricted their consumption of fruits, vegetables, pasta, and bread. What mattered was that everyone, it seemed, knew someone who had been on a low-carbohydrate diet and raved about it, proudly proclaiming that they had easily, effortlessly, lost weight.

Meanwhile, nutritionists were still warning that a calorie is a calorie and low-carbohydrate diets could be dangerous to your health.

And a few academic researchers were warning that the constant blame-the-victim message, the notion that anyone could be thin if they really wanted to or if they found the right diet, was not only demoralizing fat people but leading to a society in which prejudice against the overweight and obese has become the last remaining socially acceptable one. Telling fat people that substantial weight loss was imperative, as nutritionists and public health groups and physicians did, and telling them that there was a diet that would make them thin, as Atkins and other diet promoters did, was not helpful.

"Obese people get a level of abuse now that could not even be considered with any other group," says Jeffrey Friedman, an obesity researcher at Rockefeller University. Looking like a stereotypical rumpled scientist, long and lanky with no significant weight problem, Friedman is speaking not from personal experience but from his own research that showed him that sustained and substantial weight loss is problematic for nearly everyone. And he despairs over the plight of fat people.

"We have this naïve view that the whole system of weight control can be controlled by willpower," Friedman says. He likes to cite weight loss advice from two millennia ago—eat less and exercise more. "We have to do better than repeating two-thousand-year-old mantras," he says.

But Jeff Friedman's audience is mostly scientists. Most constant dieters, like Carmen Pirollo, have never heard of him. And as for those academic arguments about low-carbohydrate versus low-calorie, they were, Carmen thought, well, academic, and he was dimly aware of them at best. With a diet history that encapsulated the weight loss fads of the late twentieth century, his story was a prime example of the endless odyssey that sends most dieters from one popular program to another, looking for that mythical diet to end all diets, the diet that will rid them of their excess weight once and for all.

Carmen found out about the Penn study in January 2004 when he read a column in *The Philadelphia Inquirer* saying the University of Pennsylvania was seeking obese men, in particular, to be study subjects. (The study was supposed to include equal numbers of men and women, but it can be particularly hard to sign up men because they tend to be less likely to join organized weight loss programs. The researchers ended up with about two hundred women and one hundred men.)

"I put the article down and called within thirty seconds," he said. It was, he thought, his last best hope. This program would be something different, supervised by researchers at a leading medical center, and it would entail a responsibility, a *pledge*, to keep coming back for two years, a commitment to being tested, being weighed, coming to meetings with a small group of fellow dieters. Once he began, Carmen decided, the program would be more than a diet. The program would be a promise to science, and it would be almost impossible to drop out. He could barely wait to start. He was at a point of desperation. He had known what it was like to be thin, and he wanted to return to that world.

The weight had crept up on Carmen over his adult lifetime. "I was skinny as a twig until right after college, as were my father and grandparents before me," he says. "It wasn't a matter of my being a jock or anything in high school and college. I wasn't on any sports teams," so it was not as if he suddenly went from an active life to a sedentary one. He suspects his weight gain was determined by his genes.

"From the time I was twenty-four or twenty-five, I started to put on weight. It was all incremental. I had been 165 in college; then I went to 180. I thought that was enormously fat. Then I went to 200, and I thought that was enormously fat. When I was thirty, I weighed 210, and I thought that was enormously fat." But even though he's reached 265 pounds, he does not look lumberingly heavy, and he knows it. "That was really something that got me into a lot of trouble. People would say, 'You're not fat,' so I could have another portion of what I was eating. For me, and for a lot of men, it all ends up in front. I've got the rear end in front. Believe me, it is there."

He tried repeatedly to lose weight and keep it off, starting with fad diets—the grapefruit diet, the hard-boiled egg diet, "everything that came down the pike." He called them "water-cooler diets." They are, he says, the thing you talk about at the water cooler, and that is how they spread from person to person. But they were of little help. Each time, he would lose 10 or 15 pounds, then gain them back. Carmen still has those old diets—he keeps the sheets of instructions for them in a folder in his basement the same way another person might keep old yearbooks or diaries. Each one brings back memories, like hearing an old song or smelling an aroma from your past. If he looked at an old diet, the sensations came flooding back—that wonderful feeling of iron discipline, of self-control. The giddy thrill of watching the numbers on the scale plunge. And the period of regaining that weight? It was never part of the fond memories evoked by the diet sheets. The weight gain was separate from the diet, a sign of weakness or a lack of resolve, not a problem with the diet.

Over the years, as his weight inched up, Carmen began to worry about the health consequences of being fat. His father was a diabetic and had died of heart disease, and his uncle, his father's younger brother, had died of heart disease. "I just thought, Let me diet so I don't become diabetic," Carmen says. And, of course, he is concerned about his appearance. "I'm an American. We live in a society where people have to be beautiful."

In 1996, at age forty-two and weighing 218 pounds, he decided it was time to try something different from those self-help water-cooler diets. What he needed was a national diet program, something you pay to join. He considered Weight Watchers, but concluded that it was not for him. Carmen lives alone in Center City Philadelphia, a vibrant area of the city, with his two dogs, Buddy and Butch, and does not enjoy preparing food. Even if he did, he insists, he would never want to be on a Weight Watchers type of diet, weighing and measuring his food, recording every bite he ate, and exerting excruciating control over his portion sizes. A better option, he decided, would be Jenny Craig, where all the work is done for you. Each week he would be given his food, every meal prepackaged, already weighed and measured. It seemed easy.

"Talk about portion control," Carmen says. "Initially, you look at it and think you will starve to death. But you do acclimate to it. Being a good Catholic boy from the old days, I had no problem with regimentation." He told his counselor at Jenny Craig that he wanted to weigh 165, and managed to get there, dieting himself to true skinniness, so much so that some of his friends and colleagues at work were concerned. "Oh, I made it," Carmen says. "People thought I was sick." His Jenny Craig center even wanted to hire him to work part-time as a counselor and, of course, role model for all their clients who wondered if the system was really going to make them lose weight.

But within a year after Carmen left Jenny Craig, all the pounds he lost had come back, and more. Despairing, he noticed that a custodian at his school who had always been fat was dropping pounds, fast. What, Carmen asked him, was the secret? "He said he had a doctor, a very legitimate doctor in Philadelphia, who had this new magic pill."

Carmen called and made an appointment with the custodian's doctor. The pill turned out to be phen-fen, for phentermine-fenfluramine. It was a combination of an appetite suppressant (phentermine) and a drug that not only tamped down appetite but also slightly increased the metabolic rate (fenfluramine), and it was a drug treatment that was sweeping the nation. Doctors and patients were saying that this was the only diet pill they had seen that actually worked. Doctors were setting up phen-fen mills. It worked for Carmen, too; he says the weight came off effortlessly. Every week he went to the doctor, and every time the routine was the same. "I had a B12 shot, I was weighed, I got the pills. Then out you go. It was costly, but you just lose weight. I don't remember suffering in the slightest and I'd say I lost 20, 25 pounds."

Carmen, it turned out, was coming in at the end of one of the great cautionary tales in the annals of weight loss in the twentieth century.

The story began more than two decades ago when phentermine and fenfluramine were approved for short-term use as diet aids. They never gained much of a market because they were not very effective. But in 1979, Michael Weintraub, a professor of clinical pharmacology at the University of Rochester, got the idea of trying them in combination.

His inspiration was that maybe two mediocre weight loss drugs, with different actions on the brain, might complement each other to give a powerful, long-lasting effect. So he decided to enroll overweight people in a study, giving them the drugs along with intensive help with diet, exercise, and behavior modification. If it worked and the study subjects lost weight, he would not simply send them back to their old ways. Instead, he decided, he would consider obesity to be a chronic disease, like diabetes or high blood pressure, and encourage people to take the drugs to get their weight down and then continue taking the drugs for the rest of their lives to keep their weight under control.

That was the start of a four-year study of 121 obese people, mostly women, with an average weight of 200 pounds. They alternately took phen-fen or placebos. Weintraub noticed that when his subjects were taking placebos, they said they were always hungry and gained weight; when they took phen-fen, their appetites diminished and their weight dropped. At the end of the study, the participants had lost an average of 30 pounds, an astonishing success in a field that had known so few.

Weintraub assumed the drugs were safe. "I figured, gee whiz, these drugs have been on the market for ten, twelve years. Everything must be known about them." He could hardly wait to tell the world about the regimen's success over four years, something no drug, no diet, had ever before accomplished. But medical journals were not interested in publishing his paper. He thought he knew why. "Journals were loath to print articles extolling the benefits of drug therapy."

Finally, in July 1992, the work appeared in *Clinical Pharmacology & Therapeutics*. It was not a well-known journal and hardly on the medical profession's must-read list. But it was noticed by the media—which received a press release from the University of Rochester—and then by doctors and patients. And the floodgates were opened.

Ben Z. Krentzman, a family practitioner, saw a newspaper article about the study and came out of retirement to prescribe the pills. He began by advertising on the Internet and seeing patients in his living room. Soon, he opened an office in Culver City, California, and then he opened two more—one in San Luis Obispo, California, and the other in Hawaii. By 1997, he reported that he had given the drugs to eight hundred people.

Pietr Hitzig, a doctor in Timonium, Maryland, said he gave the pills to eight thousand people and advertised on his Web page that if you could not make it to his office, he would prescribe the drugs anyway over the phone. There are no contraindications, his Web page said.

Dennis Tison, a Sacramento psychiatrist, soon found himself doing nothing but dispensing phen-fen. He bought the drugs wholesale and sold them in his office to thousands of patients, advertising his services on the Internet. "I got calls from all over the country," he said. "People would say, 'I want the meds and I will pay anything.'"

His practice, Tison said, was nothing like the storefront clinics springing up overnight in California strip malls "like cockroaches," handing out the drugs to anyone who walked in. "A lot of doctors viewed this as a cash register," Tison complained.

Commercial weight loss centers also gave out the drugs. One, California Medical Weight Loss Associates, which had sixteen offices in the Los Angeles area, gave phen-fen to about ten thousand people. "This is L.A.," said Aaron Baumann, the group's administrator. "People tend to want to be thinner than in the rest of the country." He said the drugs "work like magic." He himself took them.

Jenny Craig provided phen-fen to clients, and NutriSystem advertised two months of free medication with either phen-fen or dexfenfluramine to dieters who switched to them from Jenny Craig.

The Internet bristled with phen-fen advertisements, including one that rather mysteriously quoted "L.D., San Diego" as saying, "I lost 40 pounds in six weeks on phen-fen and had to force myself to eat."

The Web page added, "It was so easy," and promised to tell more for five dollars.

It was not just the obese who took the drugs. Many doctors, including Hitzig and Krentzman, prescribed them to people with just a few pounds to lose. Hitzig's Web page quoted a patient saying that until taking phen-fen, "no matter what I did, I could never shed that last 15 pounds." Hitzig also prescribed the drugs for people with eating disorders, who may not be overweight, as well as for alcoholics, cocaine addicts, and people complaining of Gulf War syndrome. His idea was that if they worked for overeating—and overeating, he had decided, was an addiction—then they should work for other addictions, too. Gulf War syndrome might seem like a stretch, but if the drugs worked, they worked, Hitzig decided. But the vast majority of his patients wanted to lose weight.

Baumann, of California Medical Weight Loss Associates, said that doctors there prescribed the pills for people who were at least 20 percent above their ideal weight. "A lady who weighs 120 and should weigh 100 pounds is obese," he said, conceding, however, that "you might not look at her and say she is obese."

Even university medical centers, including the one at the University of Pennsylvania, where Carmen enrolled in the Atkins versus low-calorie diet study, prescribed phen-fen.

In 1996 alone, doctors across the country wrote eighteen million prescriptions for the drugs.

Weintraub watched the roaring phen-fen fad with increasing astonishment and dismay, saying he was appalled by what he had wrought, taken aback by the phen-fen industry. "In truth, I never thought of phen-fen mills," he said, reflecting on the phenomenon five years after his paper was published. "I never thought of it as a magic pill—every time I hear that word, I sort of cringe."

The end came soon. In July 1997, while Carmen, blissfully unaware of any concerns, was happily losing weight, doctors at the Mayo Clinic in Rochester, Minnesota, reported that twenty-four women taking fenfluramine or dexfenfluramine became ill with a rare and gravely serious heart valve abnormality.

Wyeth-Ayerst (now known as Wyeth), one of two companies that made fenfluramine and the sole maker of dexfenfluramine, a newer version of the drug, which it sold as Redux, sent out a news release saying it was working with the Mayo Clinic to further investigate the question of whether phen-fen caused the heart valve defects but added that so far the data were "limited and therefore not conclusive." In addition, said the company, the drugs might be promoting better health because obesity itself "is associated with serious health disorders."

The Food and Drug Administration (FDA) asked doctors across the country to report patients with similar valve damage and soon accumulated more than a hundred cases. A few months later, five medical centers independently told the FDA that they had done echocardiograms on 291 patients, mostly women, taking one of the two drugs and saw that a third of them had damaged aortic or mitral valves, though none had symptoms of heart damage, such as tiredness or shortness of breath. The drugs were removed from the market.

It was not clear whether the drugs were to blame for the heart valve problems. The symptoms of valve defects are common—tiring easily or becoming breathless with little exertion—and if people are told they might have those symptoms, many notice that they do. The problem was that no one knew the percentage of the general population with valve damage, and so it was difficult to decide whether there was an unusual increase in incidence in people taking phen-fen. But by mid-September 1997, when the drugs were withdrawn, lawyers were actively recruiting patients for lawsuits against Wyeth. And Wyeth, while denying that the drugs had caused a medical disaster, ended up setting aside nearly $17 billion to cover its liability.

Carmen, like millions of others, stopped taking the drugs. He was worried and angry that his health might have been endangered. "When I was nine years old, I had a heart murmur," he said. Might that have made him vulnerable to a terrible side effect of the drugs? Soon, he was bombarded with letters and calls from lawyers—he says he has no idea how they found him. "They were relentless. They would not let you *not* be part of their lawsuit. As there was a bumper crop of physicians giving out the drugs, now there was a bumper crop of lawyers. I was getting this from every law office in the world."

He signed up with Marvin Lundy, a personal injury lawyer with offices in the Philadelphia area, who sent him to a hotel near the Philadelphia airport for testing. The law office had rented two rooms, had set up an echocardiogram, and was screening a lineup of former phen-fen patients. "One by one, we were called in," Carmen said. Then nothing. No word on whether the test had found valve damage. No money. He called Lundy's office and was told they were backed up trying to assess all the test results. In the meantime, he said, Lundy sent him birthday cards and Christmas cards. Finally, in May 2003, Carmen got a letter from the law firm. "It said, 'Here are the results. Everything is fine with your heart. Goodbye and good luck.' I called and said, 'Aren't you forgetting about long-range problems?'" But he was politely dismissed. "No more Christmas cards from Marvin Lundy," Carmen says.

Without phen-fen, Carmen was at a loss to control his weight. "I stopped, and the weight came back," he recalls. What to do? He had no interest in trying another water-cooler diet, so, like the swallows of Capistrano who, legend has it, return each year to an old ruined church where they had been saved in the past from an innkeeper who destroyed their nest, Carmen returned to Jenny Craig. It was the only weight loss regimen other than phen-fen that had really gotten his weight down, and he hoped the program might work its charm on him again. But this time, in 1998, the magic was gone, and he could not get into the rhythm and regimen of the program. "I found that after two months I pretty much gave it up."

In January 2003, he finally tried the Atkins diet. It was a last resort, something he had been resisting. He had been hearing about it for years and some of his friends had lost weight with it, but Carmen had said no, it was not for him. "I looked at it and said, 'I could never do that. I love my potato chips. I love my pasta.' After all, I'm Italian. And Atkins did not have a good name. It was for all intents and purposes a fad diet. It was going to build up your cholesterol, give you a heart attack, give you a stroke."

But suddenly the diet became wildly popular, and Carmen had the impression that doctors were no longer quite so adamant that it was bad for your health. So he went to a bookstore and picked up Atkins's book *Dr. Atkins' New Diet Revolution*, hoping against hope that it would not include what he thought of as "that dreaded weighing and measuring thing." By page 28, he knew it was the diet for him. It told him what to eat and what to avoid. And he would not have to weigh and measure—carefully controlled portion sizes were definitely not part of the diet plan. "It goes back to my upbringing as a Catholic boy—'no meat on Friday' and 'this is what you must do.' That's what I need. And there it was. Here is what I was allowed to eat. Here is what I was not allowed to eat."

He started the diet. It was his New Year's resolution—stay on the diet, lose the weight. "I was amazed at how quickly the weight was coming off. I lost 9 or 10 pounds in the first week. I took it with a grain of salt because I know we slosh a lot of water around in our bodies. You lose a lot of water weight, and then, once you purge yourself of toxins, it is, like, 3 or 4 pounds a week, then it's, like, 1 or 2 pounds." Yet he was not hungry; his food cravings had vanished; his acid reflux was gone; even his cholesterol level went down. Before he knew it, he had lost 40 pounds and weighed just 210.

Carmen loved his new body. "You walk down the street and say, *Hey*, I look *good*. And I'm probably healthy." He could not imagine getting fat again.

Then he began to backslide. "This is how it started. It was summer, and there were beautiful strawberries and beautiful blueberries. Those are the only fruits you can have on the diet, and I would put them in a bowl of cream. But then there were Jersey peaches and beautiful Jersey tomatoes. Summer was here. The harvest was in. I was my own master, and I thought, Well, those are natural, God-given foods. They can't be too much of a problem. But they were. Then you get into having the bun with the hamburger. I returned to pasta and breads, all kinds of grains came back. By September, as every teacher will tell you, we get very depressed. I was rewarding myself with food, as I always did. Then I knew, Oh, it's coming back." And it did. "Forty pounds came back within six months."

It seemed almost an omen when Carmen found out about the University of Pennsylvania study comparing the Atkins diet with the low-calorie one. It was January again, time for a new start, time to repeat the old diet magic. It seemed fated. "I had the willies," Carmen says. To his dismay, however, he had to take a battery of physical and psychological tests that dragged on, lasting until the meeting on March 1.

"I had that mentality—Gee, last time I started in January. Now I'm starting in March. I'm going to be as thin in June as I was in April." He and the others were growing increasingly impatient. "We were all saying, 'When do we start? When do we start?'"

In the meantime, Carmen's weight was climbing. "I said, 'I know what I'm going into, and I know it will be rigorous. So I'm having ice cream tonight. And this is my last hamburger.' I wanted to be sure I tasted everything I could, from Tastykake blueberry pie to ice cream. Potato chips, everything, so I could say goodbye to it."

He knew that he might be assigned to the low-calorie diet, with all that weighing and measuring of food, and he prayed it would not happen.

"I was worried. I was truly worried that I was not going to be on Atkins. I tried in every way I could to let it be known. I said, 'If you're looking for success at the end of two years . . .'; I said, 'If you have one thousand people and three hundred drop out, I truly do not want to be one of those people.'" In the self-evaluations he did before the study began, he told the researchers again how much he wanted the Atkins diet. "I put that in quite a few times. I was telling them right out that Atkins was my way to go and I had done it before."

Of course, the researchers did not hand-pick subjects for one diet or another—the diet choice was made at random, and Carmen had a fifty-fifty chance of getting the diet he wanted. He won—he was assigned to the Atkins diet. "I was very lucky," he says. "In truth, if it had gone the other way, not being a cook, not being a food shopper, I would have been depressed and disappointed."

He was determined to succeed, to lose the weight this time and keep it off for life. "If it doesn't work, if this Atkins component with every bit of support doesn't work, then there's something wrong with me."

On March 1, Carmen sat at a long, narrow white table in a windowless white room on the third floor of an office building where the University of Pennsylvania rents space. It was five-thirty on a damp, gray evening, the end of a long, cold winter, and this was the first formal meeting of a group of Atkins diet subjects who had passed all the preliminary screening tests and who understood that they, these eight men and one woman, were expected to show up in this stark, unadorned room for one hour on Monday nights for the next two years. If they had to be absent, they were to notify the group facilitators in advance. Now the study was going to get under way in earnest. Now there was no backing down.

When Carmen entered the room, he sat in what was to be his regular spot—there were no assigned seats, but each person took a place that first night and claimed it, sitting in the same chair at every meeting from then on. Carmen's seat was near the head of the table, where the facilitators were sitting. They were two slender, pretty young women—Leslie Womble and Eva Epstein—who looked as if they had never had to worry about their weight. Leslie, who has a Ph.D. in clinical psychology, was the group leader, and Eva, working toward a Ph.D. in clinical psychology at nearby Temple University, was Leslie's assistant.

Leslie was a warm blonde. The mother of a toddler, she was soon to become pregnant with a second little girl. She had a calm and soothing demeanor, exuding understanding and a sort of tough love. Eva was more the college student, unmarried, her dark hair pulled back. She had more of an eager look, ready to nod and smile and show with her every move how much she wanted to help the struggling dieters. Leslie and Eva's role was not to tell the dieters what to do so much as to ask questions. How does that make you feel? What else might you do to distract yourself from your urge to eat? How many of you kept food diaries this week? But never, absolutely never, did they recite the dieters' weight gains and losses. That was private information because this, after all, was not a diet contest.

As the first meeting began, all the participants, in turn, told why they were there and what they hoped to accomplish. It was a litany of failed attempts at weight control—half the people in the room had even tried the Atkins diet, only to gain the weight back again.

A retired man was first to speak. "I have a lifetime of losing weight. I do it well, but then I gain it back. I really feel my weight management sucks." A younger man reported that he had been on and off diets for at least fifteen years. "I am looking forward to participating and learning some techniques to change my philosophy, my behavior." A middle-aged man said he had always been heavy and had long battled an addiction to cigarettes. "I would stop smoking, gain weight, start again." But he would fail to lose the weight he had just gained. With every gain-loss cycle, he said, his weight would click up another notch.

Forty-five minutes ticked by, the dismal diet histories all starting to sound alike. Finally, everyone had spoken, all the sorry stories had been aired.

Okay, Carmen thought. Now we will start the diet. He was more than ready, feeling if anything a bit ill from all the foods he'd been saying goodbye to. He was ready for a nice strict spartan regimen, ready to feel cleansed of all of his eating sins. But no. The diet was not to start that week, the group leader, Leslie, told them. She carefully explained to the crestfallen subjects that they had to take the coming week to prepare for the diet. They had to purge their houses of forbidden foods. They had to shop for the low-carbohydrate foods they would need. They had to keep a food diary of what they were eating, and when. They had to get psychologically ready. Then, and only then, would the diet begin.

carbohydrates was raising insulin levels, causing diabetes. And the more insulin in your blood, the more you will lay down fat. No wonder people are getting fatter and fatter, no wonder so many are despairing about getting their weight under control.

The hypothesis was presented as an exciting discovery. In fact, to have heard Robert Atkins, the late diet doctor, talk, you would think he had invented his diet. Even the names of his books stress how unique and exciting it is: *Dr. Atkins' Diet Revolution* and *Dr. Atkins' New Diet Revolution.*

But, as it turns out, nothing in the diet world is new; everything is rediscovered. It is like the world of fashion, where, women tell each other, if you save your clothes and wait long enough, they'll come into style once again.

Fashion, though, is a newcomer to the trend of endless recycling, at least when compared with diets. It turns out that when you look back at the history of diets and dieting, you notice that almost everything that people try today in their attempts to lose weight was tried as long ago as the nineteenth century. And the Atkins diet is no exception. It was first promoted by a charming French gourmet, a lawyer turned food writer who reasoned that cutting out carbohydrates was the way to lose weight.

Dieting, of course, is not the image that usually comes to mind when you think of a French gourmet or of the nineteenth century, when farmers and their families starved in lean years, when poverty and illness were so rampant that in some wards of American cities the infant mortality rate was an incredible 100 percent. But for many people of that era, dieting was a way of life. The ideal body then was quite a bit fatter than it is today. Yet still, for many, obtaining that body was an impossible dream. And the plight of the obese, derided and told it was all their own fault, was oddly familiar, their search for a way to control their weight all too poignant. Only the bluntness of the jibes has changed.

Fat men in those days told of being mocked and insulted when they went out in public. Magazines published cruel digs about the obese, like a description of a fat woman as "massive, with solid beef and streaky tallow; so that (though struggling manfully against the

2

Epiphanies and Hucksters

The Atkins diet. In the year 2004, when the Penn diet study began, it seemed that nearly everyone in the nation was on Atkins or its closely related competitor, the South Beach Diet (invented, like the Atkins diet, by a cardiologist, Arthur Agatston, director of the Mount Sinai Cardiac Prevention Center in Miami Beach, Florida), or knew someone who was on a low-carbohydrate diet or was about to try one. Atkins was more than just a diet. It was "almost like a revelation," says Rudolph Leibel, a slim and urbane obesity researcher at Columbia University who is all too familiar with the rise and fall of diets in America.

To try the diet meant doing something completely different from the tedium of weighing and measuring your meager allotment of food, or letting a company like Jenny Craig do that for you with its prepackaged diet foods, or going to those all-too-familiar group support meetings of Weight Watchers, where you start by stepping up to the scale to weigh in and where you cringe in embarrassment if your weight reveals that you've had a few diet transgressions. With Atkins you just put your faith in a sort of hand-waving scientific explanation of why calories don't count, why carbohydrates make you fat, why eating the Atkins way is the answer to your weight problems.

It seemed so logical. People had been told by all the academic experts that they had to eat less fat, and they took the advice to heart, substituting carbohydrates for fat. What a mistake that turned out to be, the Atkins types insisted. All that sugar in your blood from

idea) you inevitably think of her as made up of steaks and sirloins."
There were cruel anecdotes: "I actually knew of a lady who got wedged
between the table and bench while dining on shipboard and the car-
penter had to be sent for to saw her out. Mortifying in the extreme,
but equally ludicrous." Then there were the little rhymes. "All flesh is
grass, / the Psalmist saith. / If this be no mistake, / [When] Fat Hoyle's
cut down by death, / What loads of hay he'll make."

And just as today, when thinness is more of an obsession for
women than for men and more a concern for the rich than for the
poor, so it was in the nineteenth century. The differences in the nineteenth century, though, were a bit more pronounced. Many immi-
grants, particularly those from Germany, as well as actresses and
prostitutes, were plump, and wanted to stay that way. So did some
fat men, who cultivated their heft as part of their power. It was the
age of businessman James Buchanan Brady, or "Diamond Jim," who
was as famous for eating huge, luxurious meals as he was for his col-
lection of diamonds and jewels and his enormous wealth, estimated
at $10 to $20 million when he died in his sleep in 1917, at age sixty-
one, of a heart attack. And it was an age when some proudly portly
men joined "Fat Men's Clubs" in the United States and England.

Women who were entertainers, like British music hall stars who
performed in America, were held to very different standards than
the wan and thin women of the upper class. These music hall performers were derided as "beefy" but remained popular, admired by
men for their voluptuousness. One of the great beauties of the time,
stage star Lillian Russell, weighed about 200 pounds. And Russell,
known as "airy, fairy Lillian, the American Beauty," had a legendary
appetite, notes historian Harvey Levenstein of McMaster University
in Ontario, Canada—so huge that it came as a shock to one of her
great admirers.

Levenstein relates the story of Oscar Tschirky, or Oscar of the
Waldorf, a Swiss immigrant who became headwaiter at the Waldorf
Hotel, working there for fifty years and presenting to the world
eggs Benedict, Waldorf salad, and Thousand Island dressing. Before
he arrived at the Waldorf in 1893, Levenstein reports, Tschirky
worked at Delmonico's Restaurant, taking the job "largely because
Russell, whom he worshiped from afar, dined there three or four
times a week." He goes on: "Finally placed in charge of the private

dining rooms, he at last had his chance to serve her while she dined with Diamond Jim Brady, who also had an impressive appetite. Alas, Tschirky later told his biographer, 'I had the surprise and disillusionment of a lifetime. Lillian Russell ate more than Diamond Jim.'"

Upper-class women, though, were a different story. Fashion decreed that they be thin enough to have an 18-inch corseted waist, so narrow that a man could span it with his hands. Far from being gourmands, these women were more like invalids, and lower-class American women who married into the upper classes quickly learned to adapt. They would corset themselves and feign illness because frailty was part of the much-desired image. Lois Banner, a professor of history at the University of Southern California, tells of a former bareback rider in the circus, Josephine DeMott, who married a rich man from Cincinnati and adapted to her new status: "She laced her corsets to eighteen inches and then carefully became ill all the time, as were most of the women in her new circle. She bought herself an expensive cut-glass smelling-salts bottle topped by a diamond that she carried to revive her after her fainting attacks. She visited doctors and discussed her medical problems with all her friends. 'It was a thrilling game.'"

The problem then, as now, came for those who just could not force their bodies into the beauty standards of the day. Many struggled mightily with their personal body projects, hoping to control their weight and, all too often, lurching from success to relapse. It was the perfect setting for promoters of diets. And so they emerged.

Of course, dieting did not start with the nineteenth century. There is no real starting point for dieting, no date when it became clear that men and women were depriving themselves of food they craved because they wanted to look better or regain their health. Diets date back to at least the time of the ancient Greeks, and as long as people were writing their memoirs, there were those who could not resist describing the hoary tale of redemption through weight loss. Fat, in the European tradition, was a sign of gluttony. Gluttony was a sin, dieting almost a rite of purification.

But the nineteenth century was different, and in a sense, that difference emerged with the first incarnation of the Atkins diet.

It began with a French lawyer, Jean Anthelme Brillat-Savarin, who instructed his devotees in his international bestseller *The Phys-*

iology of Taste, one of the most famous books ever written about food. In his book, which he wrote and self-published in 1825, Brillat-Savarin warned about diet fads and, in particular, about drinking vinegar to lose weight. That was a remedy as popular in the United States as it was in Europe—it was the nineteenth century's version of the diet supplement ephedra. And, like ephedra, the vinegar prescription had doctors wringing their hands and dieters seeking it out for what they hoped would be its miraculous properties. It had been popularized by a celebrity, Lord Byron, the British poet who was sort of the Elvis of his day and who ushered in the century with his unceasing struggles with his weight. Byron was so admired, so imitated, that his bizarre weight-control methods took hold in the United States as well as in Europe and remained popular not only during his lifetime but long after his death.

Byron's constant battle with creeping pudginess—he inherited his tendency to plumpness from his obese mother, he said—was of never-ending fascination to his fans and critics in Europe and America. And nearly everyone who despaired over how hard it is to lose weight understood his lament that everything he ate turned to fat on his body.

Edward John Trelawny, a fierce competitor of Byron's, wrote, "Byron had not damaged his body by strong drinks, but his terror of getting fat was so great that he reduced his diet to the point of absolute starvation. He said everything he swallowed was instantly converted into tallow and deposited on his ribs." Byron, he added, "was always hungry," and when he gave in and ate, he instantly gained weight.

Byron's diets were legendary—one raisin and a glass of brandy a day, or a mess of greens doused in vinegar. He'd stave off hunger pangs with tobacco and green tea. And, over and over again, he resorted to drinking vinegar.

Historian Lois Banner notes, "The popularity of drinking vinegar to lose weight can be traced directly to Byron, whose most popular regimen, according to some accounts, was to subsist for some days on vinegar and water."

Brillat-Savarin told a cautionary tale about vinegar diets in his book. Don't try it, he warned, or you may have the same tragic fate as a young woman he loved when he was just twenty years old.

Her name was Louise and she was pleasingly plump, and Brillat-Savarin was simply smitten, writing in *The Physiology of Taste* that she was one of the loveliest people he had ever known. One evening, he noticed that she seemed a bit thinner than before and asked if she was ill.

"Not at all," she replied with a smile that had something melancholy about it. "I feel perfectly well, and if by chance I have lost a little weight, I really would not miss it." But her weight continued to drop, "her cheeks became hollow," and finally, one evening, Brillat-Savarin persuaded her to tell him what was happening. She confessed that her friends had been taunting her about her weight and she had sought counsel on how to drop those unwanted pounds. The advice, which she followed, was to drink a glass of vinegar every morning. "She added that until that moment she had told no one of her program."

Brillat-Savarin was alarmed and told Louise's mother, but to no avail. The damage was done. She died in his arms, he related. "The lovely Louise went to sleep for all eternity when she was but barely eighteen years old."

How, then, should you lose weight? Brillat-Savarin had a method, he told his readers. He himself had a weight problem, he confessed, writing that he had a "fairly prominent stomach." He added, "I have always looked on my paunch as a redoubtable enemy; I have conquered it and limited its outlines to the purely majestic; but in order to win the fight I have fought hard indeed; what is good about the results and my present observations I owe to a thirty-year battle."

But like fat people today, he blamed himself. While some are more prone to obesity than others, he declared, "if obesity is not actually a disease, it is at least a most unpleasant state of ill health and one into which we almost always fall because of our own fault."

And what, he asked, do people do to keep themselves fat? He had noticed a particular pattern. His many fat dinner companions over the years indulged themselves with potatoes and rice, with breads and rich desserts. He described typical dialogues over dinner with his plump friends. A "Fat Lady," for example, exclaimed, "Nothing delights me more than pastry. We have a pastry cook as one of our tenants, and, between my daughter and myself, I truly believe that we eat up the price of his rent, and a little more besides."

Observations like that, he said, led him to what he called "an infallible system." He had noticed that carnivorous animals do not grow fat, nor do herbivores, unless they are fed grain specifically to fatten them. Starches and grains, he reasoned, are making people fat, along with an unfortunate tendency to eat not from hunger but simply because something tastes good. "It has rightly been said that one of the privileges of the human race is to eat without hunger and drink without thirst," he wrote. The problem with civilized humans is that "we eat too much." The solution to obesity, he advised, requires "a more or less rigid abstinence from everything that is starchy or floury," and, in particular, sugar mixed with flour.

He knew what sort of response that would get:

"Oh Heavens!" all you readers of both sexes will cry out, "oh Heavens above! But what a wretch the Professor is! Here in a single word he forbids us everything we must love, those little white rolls from Limet, and Achard's cakes, and those cookies from . . . , and a hundred things made with flour and butter, with flour and sugar, with flour and sugar and eggs! He doesn't even leave us potatoes or macaroni! Who would have thought this of a lover of good food who seemed so pleasant?"

"What's this I hear?" I exclaim, putting on my severest face, which I do perhaps once a year. "Very well then; eat! Get fat! Become ugly and thick, and asthmatic, finally die in your own melted grease."

Yet not everyone is ready to change his ways, Brillat-Savarin confessed: "M. Louis Greffulhe, who was later honored by His Majesty with the title of count, came to see me one morning, and told me he understood I was interested in the subject of obesity, and that since he was in grave danger of it, he wished my advice."

Brillat-Savarin said he would be happy to help, but Greffulhe must promise to do exactly as he said for one month. The man agreed, returning a month later, thinner but miserable, explaining,

Sir, I have followed your prescriptions as faithfully as if my life depended upon it, and I have verified the fact that my weight has gone down by some three pounds, or even a little

bit more. But, in order to achieve this, I have been forced to
submit all my tastes and all my habits to such a violent assault,
and in a word I have suffered so much, that while I offer you
all my thanks for your excellent advice, I must renounce what
good it might do for me, and abandon myself to whatever
Providence has in store for me.

He got fatter and fatter, and finally died, at age forty, "as the result of an asthmatic condition to which he had become subject."

But while Brillat-Savarin's book was popular, it was a few decades
before his diet took off. Perhaps this was because he never really got
rid of his paunch, even though he said he adhered to his high-
protein diet. Or perhaps it was because he died shortly after his book
appeared and so could not offer the sort of personal testimonials that
make a diet popular. But, for whatever reason, his diet came into its
own only after it was rediscovered by a London undertaker, William
Banting, who told the world about how the diet had changed his life,
freeing him from the tortures of obesity. When the diet was rediscovered in 1863, it became so trendy that, for years, the word for
dieting became "banting," after the undertaker who went on the diet.

Banting told his story in a surprise international bestseller, a
pamphlet called *Letter on Corpulence*, which follows the traditional
form of dietary evangelism. He was lost and then he was found, and
the solution to his problem was a wondrous diet that truly transformed his life.

Banting's life was ruined by his obesity. He had gotten enormously
fat, *gargantuan*, and he could not understand why. No one on either
side of his family was overweight; he himself had led an active life
and, he said, he did not really eat too much, "except that I partook
of the simple aliments of bread, milk, butter, beer, sugar, and potatoes more freely than my age required." He was thirty when his weight
started to rise, and he tried his best to control it, asking a doctor
what to do. The advice was to exercise, so he started rowing, going
out in a boat on the river for a couple of hours every morning. "It is
true I gained muscular vigor but with it a prodigious appetite, which
I was compelled to indulge, and consequently increased in weight
until my kind old friend advised me to forsake the exercise."

He asked other medical authorities for help, but no matter what he did, he got fatter and fatter: "I have tried sea air and bathing in various localities, with much walking exercise; taken gallons of physic and liquor potasse, advisedly and abundantly; adopted riding on horseback," and, over the years, "spared no trouble nor expense in consultations with the best authorities in the land, giving each and all a fair time for experiment." And, yet, he wrote, "the evil still gradually increased."

It became embarrassing for him to go out in public, where he would hear nasty remarks about his weight, the "sneers and remarks of the cruel and injudicious." By then he was truly fat, weighing 202 pounds when he was sixty-four, even though he was only 5 feet 5 inches tall. Everyday life became increasingly difficult. "I have been compelled to go down stairs slowly backwards, to save the jar of increased weight upon the ankle and knee joints, and been obliged to puff and blow with every slight exertion, particularly that of going up stairs." On top of his other ailments, Banting also was going deaf.

Finally, he found an ear, nose, and throat doctor, the eminent William Harvey, who had just come back from a medical meeting in Paris, where he had heard a talk about a new theory of diabetes which posited that the liver secretes sugar that it makes from foods people eat. In a sort of convoluted reasoning inspired by the diabetes theory, Harvey decided that Banting's loss of hearing was related to his obesity, and since diabetes often accompanies obesity, he prescribed a diet free of sugar or starch.

Banting explained,

The items from which I was advised to abstain as much as possible were: Bread, butter, milk, sugar, beer, and potatoes, which had been the main (and, I thought, innocent) elements of my subsistence, or at all events they had for many years been adopted freely. These, said my excellent adviser, contain starch and saccharine matter, tending to create fat, and should be avoided altogether. At the first blush it seemed to me that I had little left to live upon, but my kind friend soon showed me there was ample.

The diet worked. Banting said he began to feel better almost immediately, and within a year he had lost 50 pounds. He knew he was still a little plump, but he was happy with his thinner body and vastly improved health. A hernia got better on its own; his sight and hearing, he wrote, "are surprising for my age," adding, "My other bodily ailments have become mere matters of history."

Eternally grateful to Harvey, he not only paid him his usual fee but gave him another fifty pounds to give to his favorite hospitals. "I am most thankful to Almighty Providence for mercies received, and determined still to press the case into public notice as a token of gratitude," Banting wrote. "I am fully persuaded that thousands of our fellow-men might profit equally by a similar course to mine; but, constitutions not being all alike, a different course of treatment may be advisable for the removal of so tormenting an affliction."

He gave away the first two thousand copies of his pamphlet to medical authorities and the public and then watched in amazement as fifty thousand copies were sold in the first eight months of publication. The pamphlet went through twelve editions from 1863 to 1902.

Like diet promoters today, Banting was met with a mixture of awe and derision. Some said there is nothing magical about the diet—it is not the lack of carbohydrates that makes people lose weight but the paucity of food. "It is easy to become thin by not taking sufficient food," sniffed the London *Standard* in 1884, a time when Banting's diet was the most popular weight-reducing scheme in America.

Others criticized Harvey's complicity with what they saw as Banting's real motive in his quest to lose weight. "It is the business of a doctor to cure disease, not to minister to personal vanity," wrote an Edinburgh magazine, *Blackwood's*, in 1864, in an article widely read and reprinted, including by a weekly magazine in the United States.

Moreover, the magazine chided, Banting's diet is hardly new. "The system recommended by Savarin is, as our readers will observe, in essentials the same as that which Mr. Banting has proclaimed, with so much pomposity, to be an original discovery," it said, but Brillat-Savarin's description of it was "infinitely more elegant and refined." Yet, the magazine argued, the hypothesis that carbohydrates are what makes people fat is not substantiated, at least by Banting:

> We rise from the perusal of Mr. Banting's pamphlet with our belief quite unshaken in the value of bread and potatoes as ordinary and universal articles of diet. We maintain the excel-

lency and innocencey of porridge and pease-pudding; and we see no reason for supposing that any one will become a Jeshurun because he uses milk with his tea, and sweetens it with a lump of sugar.

When the fourth edition of Banting's book was published—and after, he said, he had heard from eighteen hundred readers—he wrote a preface defending himself against his critics. His correspondents were eternally grateful to him for providing the diet: "There is scarcely one out of the whole which does not breathe a spirit of pure thankfulness and gratitude for the benefits derived from the dietary system." And he was stung by the vitriol of those who derided him: "Probably no one was ever subjected to more ridicule and abuse than I have been, in English as well as in foreign journals." The proof of the success of his approach was the testimonials he received: "I believe I have subdued my discourteous assailants by silence and patience; and I can now look with pity, not unmixed with sorrow, upon men of eminence who had the rashness and folly to designate the dietary system as 'humbug,'" Banting proclaimed.

His diet remained famous and popular, and "banting" remained synonymous with dieting. Decades later, in 1895, *The New York Times* needed to give no further explanation for the term when it published what was meant to be a humorous tale of a fat German journalist. The unfortunate man fell to the floor with a loud crash when his chair collapsed under him during a tedious meeting at the Rathaus in Hamburg. "The heavy German journalist, whose immediate injuries were not serious, has in all likelihood been asked either to resign, or to enter upon a course of banting, or to provide himself with a special chair, warranted to support a ton without creaking."

But not everyone who wanted to lose weight was banting in those days. Just as today's diets and their promoters compete for attention, with one diet waxing while another wanes, so it was in the 1800s. Some of the overweight tried eating soap, or chalk, or pickles. Some tried ipecac—which comes from the dried root of a South American shrub, *Cephaelis ipecacuanha*, and induces vomiting—or drinking camphor tea, said to suppress the appetite. People tried swallowing potassium acetate, which is a diuretic, and digitalis, which speeds up the heart.

Some tried exercise, but many said it was of little use. Banting said it only increased his appetite. Brillat-Savarin said the problem with exercise is that it is tiring, it makes you sweat, and "the whole business is hopelessly boring." Then, if anything goes wrong, if "a tiny headache is felt or an almost invisible spot shows itself on the skin, the whole system of exercise is blamed and abandoned."

And then, as now, some combined dieting with health regimens and health foods that promised more energy and vigor and a freedom from disease, a regimen that appealed to more lofty goals than assuaging people's discomfort with the shape or size of their bodies.

In the nineteenth century, the health food diet was the creation of the Reverend Sylvester Graham, for whom the graham cracker was named. His goal was moral betterment. He wanted to banish what he thought was the greatest sin, gluttony, and so he prescribed a severe diet—some said it was emaciating. His disciples became obsessed with their weight, proclaiming that their motivation was not vanity but controlling their gluttonous impulses and reaching a healthy weight.

But Graham also stressed willpower and the virtue of self-denial. He insisted that people could rise above hunger and food cravings if they would just stop being slaves to their stomachs. Eating, he emphasized, need not be controlled by mere hunger: "The whole system of governing the head by the stomach instead of governing the stomach by the head is utterly wrong. Make your stomach the healthful minister of the body, and not the whole body the mere locomotive appendage of your stomach. Treat your stomach like a well governed child; carefully find out what is best for it, as the digestive organ of your body, and then teach it to conform to your regimen."

Graham told his followers that they should eat simple foods, such as grains and vegetables, and drink water. Beef and pork, salt and pepper, spices, tea and coffee, alcohol—all led to gluttony. Bread should be unleavened, and made with bran to avoid the problem of yeast, which turned sugar into alcohol. Even holiday feasts were forbidden. Graham's close associate, the Boston health reformer William A. Alcott, decrying overindulgence, attacked feasts on Thanksgiving and the Fourth of July, and even the traditional Sunday dinners.

Graham's followers were the first Americans to keep close track of their own weight, and even to weigh their food. They wrote letters and testimonials about the power of the new way of eating, noting their weights and their new health. For example, one, John Kilton, recorded that his weight fell from 161 to 127 pounds, then rose to 146 pounds, where it remained, leaving him with "a solidity in my system that never existed there before."

Graham's method was supposed to cure people of all ills by restoring a natural diet, so his followers sought out fresh, organic fruits and vegetables, grown in soil without fertilizers, and made bran bread. They established "Physiological Boardinghouses," where people could live the Graham way. Skeptics were scathing. Dinner at a Graham house must feature such delicacies as "straggling radishes" and "a soggy bunch of asparagus," along with "corpses of potatoes" and "a thin segment of bran bread." To wash it down, these health nuts would have "a tumbler of cold water."

With their spare diet, Grahamites were known for their lean look. One satirist of the time, whose pen name was Sam Slick, wrote, "I once traveled all through the state of Maine with one of them. He was thin as a whipping post." He added that the Grahamite "put [him] in mind of a pair of kitchen tongs, all legs, shaft and head, and no belly; a real gander lookin critter, holler as a bamboo walkin cane, and twice as yeller."

It was a diet so extreme that it aroused alarm. In 1840, students and faculty at Oberlin College were made to follow Graham's diet. The experiment was abandoned a year later after some students and faculty rebelled—one student wrote, "Beware! 'There is no joking with the belly'"—and the townspeople became distressed by stories that the college's strict diet was causing mass starvation.

But Grahamism, for all the attention it got, was never really a popular movement. The next revelation, the next innovation, was very different from it or from the still-popular banting. At its heart was the idea that all you had to do to control your weight was to chew your food very, very thoroughly. That diet plan ended up supplanting the ever-popular low-carbohydrate diet and became the first diet trend of the twentieth century. The program involved not just a lot of chewing but a regimen that stressed carbohydrates, vegetarianism, and calorie-counting. And it began with an overweight, exhausted, and rich American whose weight loss method, modified a bit to make it more feasible, survives to this day in diet books and diet counseling.

The year was 1889, and forty-year-old Horace Fletcher was in despair. The wealthy businessman from Lawrence, Massachusetts, complained that his health was failing, he was always tired, and he had indigestion. He felt like "a thing fit but to be thrown on the scrapheap." Part of it was that he was fat, weighing 217 pounds even though he was only 5 feet 7 inches tall. When he applied for life insurance, he was turned down because of his excess weight. But how, he wondered, could he get thin and healthy again? Money was not an obstacle, but he needed a method, or maybe a philosophy, to guide him in life.

A decade later, he found it. Fletcher took his inspiration from a well-known and often deplored American habit of devouring food, barely taking time to chew it. As Sylvester Graham's associate William A. Alcott wrote, "We *do not* bolt our food but *throw it* down our throats." A British visitor wrote, "I never saw a Yankee that did not bolt his food whole, like a boa constrictor." Even women were virtually inhaling their food, wrote a Russian tourist: "It startles a visitor to see with what voracity even our delicate women dispose of the infinite succession of dishes on public tables."

Gulping food, Fletcher decided, was unhealthy and deprived people of the pleasure of eating. The path to healthful eating and weight control was simple, he said. Eat only when you are hungry, eat only those foods that your appetite is craving, stop when you are no longer hungry, and—the dictum for which he was most famous—chew every morsel of food until there is no more taste to be extracted from it.

As proof of his method, Fletcher gleefully recounted how his weight plummeted when he adopted his new ways. In June 1898, he weighed 205 pounds and his waist was 44 inches around. Four months later he was 42 pounds lighter, weighing 163 pounds, and had lost 7 inches around his waist. He said he also regained an amazing physical stamina. In 1897 he reported that he had tried bicycling, which had become all the rage, but found to his dismay that he was worn out by a 50-mile ride. In the summer of 1899, he is said to have ridden 100 miles with no problem. In August of that year, he is said to have surpassed even that feat. "With no special training in the interim, he celebrated his own birthday (his fiftieth!) by pedaling more than one hundred ninety miles, and was so free of fatigue and stiffness as to ride another fifty miles the next morning," writes historian James C. Whorton.

Fletcher became known as "The Great Masticator," and his followers recited and followed his instructions to chew their food one hundred times a minute. Liquids, too, had to be chewed, Fletcher insisted. But he promised that "Fletcherizing," which the technique became known as, would turn "a pitiable glutton into an intelligent epicurean." It was the origin of the idea that to be healthy, to avoid indigestion, to lose weight and to stay slim, you must eat slowly and chew thoroughly.

His fans spoke with unabashed enthusiasm. "In obtaining Fletcherism, I found myself aided greatly by being able to put only a small portion of food upon my plate when helping myself at the table. You know that we are all trained from earliest childhood to 'eat what is put before us' without question and nine persons out of ten will conscientiously finish everything put on their plates," said Goodwin Brown, a New York lawyer, in 1907. Fletcherism taught him to eat much less. Brown, writing in *The New York Times*, advocated it for everyone. Fletcherism not only improves health, but it increases attractiveness, he declared. "The good-looking man will always find his way through life to be easier than the other fellow's; and, of course, every woman wishes to look well. No woman need be fat when she practices Fletcherism, nor need she be thin—or 'skinny' as the phrase goes, for this method will bring her to her normal weight, and keep her there."

Fletcher gained celebrity endorsements. Upton Sinclair, famous for his muckraking 1906 book *The Jungle*, about the meatpacking industry, chanced upon a magazine article about Fletcher. "[It was] one of the great discoveries of my life," he declared, and went on to write a book with his friend Michael Williams, in which they extolled the Fletcher way of eating. The book's title said it all: *Good Health and How We Won It*. John D. Rockefeller was Fletcherizing. "Don't gobble your food. Fletcherize or chew very slowly when you eat," he wrote. Cookbook author and magazine columnist Sarah Tyson Rorer told her audience that they must chew each bite of food fifty times.

Some who tried the diet eventually repudiated it. Henry James, the American expatriate writer, at first embraced the program, giving out Fletcher's book, *The New Glutton*, to his neighbors and claiming that it had changed his life. He wrote to a friend, the novelist Edith Wharton, about "the divine Fletcher," and in a letter to his friend Mrs. Humphrey Ward, he waxed ecstatic: "Am I a convert, you ask? A *fanatic*." But after five years of the diet, James wrote that something awful had happened. Not only was he having stomach troubles that his doctor attributed to Fletcherism, but he found himself "more and more sickishly *loathing* food."

As his fame grew, Fletcher became a sort of Dr. Atkins of his day. Medical authorities laughed at his claims and dismissed them as blatant self-promotion. Few took seriously his insistence that he ate so little and that he no longer craved rich foods. Some who tried his diet said their lives were transformed, but others loudly proclaimed it a cruel deception, a method that almost no one could stay with for long and whose promises were largely illusionary.

In 1901, Fletcher finally managed to gain a toehold in the world of scientific credibility. In part it was because of his wealth. Research on nutrition was getting expensive, with equipment like respiration calorimeters, and was breaking scientists' budgets. "Fletcher seemed willing to devote a substantial portion of his wealth to subsidizing scientists who wished to test his theories," notes historian Harvey A. Levenstein. "When Britain's leading physiologist, Sir Michael Foster of Cambridge University, learned that Fletcher was interested in setting up a nutrition institute for research into food and physiology, he quickly invited Fletcher to Cambridge, where a few volunteers practiced chewing in the Fletcher fashion. Foster claimed to be duly impressed."

Foster and Frederick Gowland Hopkins, a professor of physiological chemistry and subsequent Nobel Prize winner, decided to put Fletcher's methods to a test. To their own astonishment, they confirmed what he had been saying. Yes, their studies lasted only a few weeks. But they never expected the results: People who Fletcherized developed appetites for simple foods, the scientists reported. They ate half what nutrition authorities had thought was necessary. And they experienced a sense of well-being and avoided constipation.

The scientists put forth a bold-faced plea for substantial support from Fletcher. It was clear, they wrote, that more research "was urgently called for," but their labs "did not possess at present either the necessary equipment or the funds to provide it." Their transparent scheme failed, however, when Fletcher hooked up instead with American scientists, who, like the British, were all too happy to use his money to pay for their research into his theories.

The American work was directed by a leading physiologist at Yale University, Russell H. Chittenden, who read the reports of the British experiments with fascination. People were eating just half what scientists thought they needed and were not ravenous or miserable? Now *that* was interesting, he thought. But, asked Chittenden, who directed Yale's Sheffield Scientific School, would the effects last if people Fletcherized for a longer period of time? He had to know, and he would start by studying Fletcher himself.

Fletcher arrived at Yale in 1902, ready to help Chittenden answer a simple question that, surprisingly, had never before been rigorously addressed. How much food *should* people eat? In Fletcher, Chittenden found what seemed like the perfect subject, someone eager to participate in an experiment on himself to discover "the smallest amount of food that will keep a body in a state of high efficiency" and someone who proclaimed that he ate very little and yet was fit and healthy. It was his chewing method, Fletcher said, that allowed him to thrive on just 1,600 calories a day. He also insisted that he ate what was thought to be a minuscule amount of protein, just 45 grams a day, about as much as is in 3 ounces of canned tuna and a cup of chickpeas. That seemingly meager portion was anathema at a time when health authorities insisted that people need 118 to 165 grams of protein a day, an idea that had come about when scientists analyzed the composition of diets eaten by people who were wealthy enough to eat whatever they wanted and who routinely consumed that much protein. (Today, the National Academy of Sciences recommends that men consume 46 grams of protein a day and women 38.)

Fletcher moved in with Chittenden, living at the professor's house for several months and showing Chittenden just how little he ate. The tiny portions were amazing, Chittenden said, but he had a different explanation for why Fletcher ate so little. It was not, as Fletcher said, because thorough chewing made digestion more efficient and detoxified foods. Instead, it was because the more you chew your food, the less food you want to eat. "To me the chewing business became unimportant except in so far as it tends to diminish the craving for food and thus results in the appetite being satisfied with a small amount. Hence to me the center of interest shifted at once to the question, how much do we really know as to the amount of food the human body requires to meet daily needs under the different conditions of life, especially protein food?"

It was becoming clear that Fletcher was thriving on his diet. When Yale's physical education expert, William G. Anderson, studied Fletcher's strength and fitness, Anderson was astonished by the middle-aged man's abilities. He put Fletcher through four days of exercises designed for Yale's crew team and reported that Fletcher performed them "with an ease that is unlooked for. He gives evidence of no soreness or lameness and the large groups of muscles respond the second day without evidence of being poisoned by carbon dioxide." In fact, Anderson said, "Mr. Fletcher performs this work with greater ease and with fewer noticeable bad results than any man of his age and condition I have ever worked with."

Fletcher said he did not make a conscious effort to restrain his eating, trusting that his method, eating only when he was hungry and engaging in what he called "divine mastication," was allowing his body to get the nutrients it needed. But Chittenden, who kept careful track of what Fletcher ate, decided that the secret of Fletcher's strength and health might lie in the small amount of protein he ate. And that led Chittenden to question the conventional nutritional advice. Was it true that most people need lots of protein? How important *was* protein? He embarked on a rigorous study that began with himself. He would become a vegetarian, or nearly so, and watch what happened.

Doctors warned him that it was risky to eat a mostly vegetarian diet, but Chittenden went ahead, inspired by the example of Horace

Fletcher. Before long, he was a convert. He lost 16 pounds, and his arthritic knees, he said, were less painful. His indigestion was relieved, his headaches less frequent, and he had gotten stronger and gained endurance.

He decided to expand the study, asking, What would be the effects of a low-protein diet on people who were sedentary, moderately active, or extremely active?

For sedentary people, or "brain workers," as he called them, he enlisted himself, his associate Lafayette Mendel, and three graduate research assistants. The extremely active were members of the varsity crew team. And for the moderately active, he found a platoon of the U.S. Army that agreed to participate.

The army was interested because, if Fletcher was correct, enlisted men would not have to be fed so much meat. So the twenty men who arrived at Yale were sent there by the army to prove that they could do fine with just a third of the normal military ration. Three of them deserted, however, and four more were thrown out of the experiment because they were caught gulping down a free lunch at a saloon nearby, which left just thirteen members of the platoon to complete the study.

From the fall of 1903 until the summer of 1904, the study participants consumed less than 15 grams of protein a day, the equivalent of one slice of cheese pizza, or half a cup of cottage cheese, or two ounces of chicken. It is an amount that, today, the National Academy of Sciences recommends for children aged four to eight. But in Chittenden's studies, no one's health declined; instead, the subjects got stronger and one athlete, the gymnast son of William Anderson, won two national championships.

Chittenden found the data so impressive that they needed little explanation:

> In presenting the results of the experiments, herein described, the writer has refrained from entering into lengthy discussions, preferring to allow the results mainly to speak for themselves. They are certainly sufficiently convincing and need no superabundance of words to give them value; indeed, such merit as the book possesses is to be found in the large number of con-

secutive results, which admit of no contradiction and need no argument to enhance their value. The results are presented as scientific facts, and the conclusions they justify are self-evident.

A few years later, Chittenden's friend Irving Fisher, an eminent Yale economist and statistician, replicated the diet experiment. He used thirty-seven Yale athletes as his subjects, assigning fifteen to eat meat and twenty-two to be vegetarians for nearly a year. The question was, Which group would be stronger? It turned out to be the vegetarians.

The tests were not quite what physiologists would require today. One was to hold your arm straight out for as long as you could. Two meat eaters, Fisher reported, could keep an arm up for more than fifteen minutes, but twenty-two out of the thirty-two vegetarians could. One of the vegetarians, in fact, managed to keep his arm extended for more than three hours.

The next test was deep knee bends. Once again, the vegetarians beat the meat eaters. The champion was a young man who did more than two thousand deep knee bends. He was a vegetarian.

"In general, it may be said that whatever the explanation, there is strong evidence that a low-proteoid, non-flesh or nearly non-flesh dietary is conducive to endurance," Fisher concluded. He remarked that the studies of low-protein diets had shown the fallacy of the widespread belief that meat-eating is needed for strength. Instead, he said, the experiments "seem gradually to be demonstrating that the fancied strength from meat is, like the fancied strength from alcohol, an illusion."

That same year, 1907, Chittenden publicized the vegetarian message again in a book, *The Nutrition of Man*, that told of his experiments and conclusions that Americans "eat too much, especially meat." *The New York Times* reviewed the book and then wrote that the publisher, Frederick A. Stokes, was deluged with orders, telling the *Times* that "no scientific book ever published by them had ever produced such an effect in so short a time." The advice was sorely needed, the *Times* scolded its readers, publishing what it said was a typical New York businessman's diet, calculating that it contained at least 3,400 calories, an amount that would be needed by a person "doing fairly active muscular work, and the average businessman does not do muscular work." To top it off, the newspaper said, there is "entirely too much proteoid" in the diet, as Chittenden's studies showed.

The more publicity the low-protein diets got, the more they raised the ire of critics, who despaired at hearing the story of Horace Fletcher as an example of the benefits of low-protein diets. How misleading, they said. Fletcher was nothing like the average person—he was endowed with extraordinary strength and stamina, and almost no human being, no matter what he ate, was going to match him.

Fletcher's boasts of his strength and endurance could become tiresome. In 1907, he informed a convention of home economists that he and the army's chief of staff, General Leonard Wood, worked for nine hours "breaking our way through the tropical jungle of a volcanic island in the Philippines." On another occasion, Fletcher told the group, he was hiking in the Himalayas, at an elevation of 8,500 feet, when he was caught in a blizzard "and was compelled to wade in deep snow for some 11 miles in nearly as many hours."

In 1908, *The Medical Record* published an article saying that Fletcher was a "somatic freak" who remained strong despite his diet, not because of it:

His endurance performances are so far ahead of anything on record as to put them outside of the normal and, as in the class of prodigies for which he is only in measure responsible; his abstemiousness and his excellent digestion dependent upon complete mastication, have not created his powers but have only developed and served to perfect the physical talents with which he was originally endowed above his fellows to an abnormal and so to say freakish degree.

The low-protein diet fad, like most other diet fads, did not last. Gradually, as people tried, and often failed to lose weight with, Fletcherism and low-protein diets, they lost their enthusiasm. By the time Fletcher died, in 1919, of a heart attack at age sixty-eight, "interest in Fletcherism was dwindling," notes historian Levenstein. Low-protein diets and thorough chewing had been supplanted by the next new thing, counting calories.

This was a dietary regimen championed by Irving Fisher, who

had concluded that calorie-counting was the only way to control your weight, and your health. With his colleague Eugene Lyman Fisk, a medical doctor, he wrote a bestselling book, *How to Live*, that explained the secret of weight loss. It is, the two wrote, to expend more calories than you consume. The mistake many make is to think that eating small amounts of food is necessarily better than eating more generous servings. That depends, the two scientists said, on the calories in the food you are eating—it is not quantity so much as calories that matters. Familiar advice today, of course, but new to people in the early twentieth century, who had not grown up with the calorie-counting mantra.

So it was a revelation when Fisher and Fisk cautioned that people often delude themselves about how much they are eating, telling themselves that "many articles such as candy, fruit, nuts and peanuts, often eaten between meals, 'do not count.'" Or when they said that people "overlook accessories, such as butter and cream, which may contain more food value than the entire meal put together." But the body is not fooled, they warned. "Nature counts every calorie very carefully. If the number of calories taken in exceeds the number used by the body (or excreted unused), the excess accumulates in fat or tissue."

They advised everyone to keep careful track of calories by using the calorie charts that their book supplied. "Constant vigilance is necessary, yet it is worthwhile when one considers the inconvenience as well as the menace of obesity," Fisher and Fisk advised their readers.

Fat people, Fisher and Fisk added, should avoid fats, sugar, milk, and a variety of meats and seafood, like sardines, mackerel, pork, and goose, as well as nuts, butter, cream, olive oil, pastry, and sweets. In the end, they say, "the reduction of weight is really a very simple matter. No mysterious or elaborate 'systems' or drugs are needed. If reduction in the amount of energy food and an increase in the amount of exercise is made, no power on earth can prevent a reduction in weight."

They called upon doctors to help. "Why do physicians take so much care measuring their dosages of drugs, which are administered only occasionally, and so little care in measuring their food prescriptions, which are administered daily?"

It was a message that fell on receptive ears. Mail-order hucksters were preying on the public's frustrating efforts to lose weight, and the federal government was urging everyone to be wary. The Department of Agriculture tested various quack weight loss remedies on its own employees to show how worthless they were. Some medications being sold were dangerous, the government warned, including drugs like thyroid hormone and laxatives and obesity remedies that included even pokeweed, a poison. Other anti-fat products had no pharmacologically active ingredients; they were the mail-order equivalent of sugar pills. One, in fact, was just a bar of soap with instructions to wash vigorously to get rid of fat. The only way to lose weight, the government insisted, was with "rigid dieting" and "strenuous exercise," and "as a general rule, diet and exercise are best directed by a skilled physician."

Soon calorie-counting was the new, preferred method for weight loss. *Eat Your Way to Health*, by a doctor, Robert H. Rose, published in 1916, said calorie-counting was "a scientific system of weight control" and that obesity was "Criminal Negligence." The next year, Herbert Hoover, who had become head of the U.S. Food Administration (later the U.S. Food and Drug Administration), announced that he was counting calories, consulting Fletcher, and using Chittenden's rules for how to do it. "I'm an engineer, and I'm not using my body," he proclaimed. "An engineer does not stoke the engine unless there is a considerable amount of power to be exerted. So I eat as little as I can to get going."

In 1918, the bestseller *Diet and Health, with Key to the Calories*, appeared, written by a physician and syndicated newspaper columnist, Lulu Hunt Peters. She dedicated her book, with permission, to Herbert Hoover. Her advice was stern: The way to get thin and stay that way was to start with a fast, to show that you are in control of your appetite, and then to Fletcherize and use Fisher and Fisk's calorie-counting methods. After the initial fast, she instructed, you must eat no more than 1,200 calories a day. When you reach your goal weight, you must go on a maintenance diet and follow it for life, always counting calories, never letting your vigilance flag, she instructed. And the need was dire. In her columns in the 1920s, Peters warned that three out of four Americans were seriously overweight.

Hotels and restaurants were quick to capitalize on the American zeal to lose weight. Even into the Great Depression, when many people were going hungry, dieting was a way of life for those with means.

Menus listed calorie counts; the Kahler hotel chain in the Midwest hired a dietician to produce calorie-counted recipes for its restaurants and cafeterias. And, notes Levenstein, "the Dessert hotel chain of the Pacific Northwest one-upped the rest. Not only did it feature the usual calorie-counted menu but its dietician had scales installed in each of its restaurants and provided a register where regular customers could keep running tabs on their weights."

But some social commentators thought all this public discussion of calories was crass. A cookbook of the era, *Food and How to Cook It*, noted that "the word 'calorie' is as familiar as the word 'food' and is heard in conversation at the luncheon table even though socially it should be taboo."

The problem was that the standards for slimness had grown stricter than ever, and more and more people felt left behind, unable to meet the new beauty requirements. Even young teenagers, who used to be less affected by dieting crazes, soon were desperately trying to lose weight. Joan Jacobs Brumberg, a Cornell University historian who studied the diaries of adolescent girls, said that before the 1920s, girls didn't write about an obsession with their weight and with dieting. That changed forever with the flapper era, when, she says, "for the first time, teenage girls made systematic efforts to lower their weight by food restriction and exercise." The new body-consciousness even emerged in popular fiction for young adolescents, Brumberg remarks. "Popular serial fiction for younger girls, such as Grace Harlow and Nancy Drew, now had a fat character who served as a humorous foil to the well-liked, smart protagonist, who was always slim."

She tells of a Chicago teenager, Yvonne Blue, whose diary in the mid-1920s "reveals how the ideal of slenderness was first incorporated into the experience of American girls."

Yvonne wrote that she wanted to be "slim and sylph-like" and that she hated herself because she was not. At age fifteen she was 5 feet 6 inches tall and weighed 150 pounds. "I am so tired of being fat," she wrote as school let out for the summer in 1926. "I'm going back to school weighing 119 pounds—I swear it. Three months in which to lose thirty pounds—but I'll do it—or die in the attempt."

She sent away for a diet book, *How to Reduce: New Waistlines for Old*, which advised consuming 1,200 to 1,500 calories a day. Yvonne tried to eat a lot less. She turned down meat and sweets and set insanely unrealistic diet goals, attempting to eat just 50 calories a day by limiting herself to lettuce, carrots, celery, tea, and consommé. She would pretend to eat to assuage her worried parents and then surreptitiously slip her food to her dog. "They *make* me eat," Yvonne complained. "Last night I dropped most of my meal in my lap and fed it to Tar Baby later." She and her friend Mattie Van Ness began dieting together—although Mattie was not fat—making a contest out of their weight loss. By the end of the summer, Yvonne weighed 125 pounds. She kept the weight off and proudly reported, at age eighteen, that she had bought a tight crêpe de chine dress that "fit like paper on the wall." She loved the saleswoman's comment: "When you are young, you should show every bump."

But despite the growing interest in calorie-counting, the allure of high-protein diets lingered and even inspired a widely publicized diet contest, akin, in those pre-television days, to the recent TV show *The Biggest Loser*.

The contest took place in New York City in 1921, directed by the city's health commissioner, Royal S. Copeland. He recruited fifty fat women who vied to see who could lose the most weight in a month. The diet? A high-protein Atkins-type one.

To great fanfare, the contest began, the diet was published, and hundreds of overweight New Yorkers tried it on their own. Compared with the spartan, low-calorie diets that were popular then, it seemed that Copeland's diet provided, if anything, too much food, but Copeland insisted that the secret was the type of food the women were eating—it was high in protein and, Copeland announced, protein is not converted to fat. He advised women what to eat: "Have it clear in your mind the kind of food you can eat freely and the kind you ought not to eat at all. Here is one girl who confessed to me freely that on Friday they had some nice, fresh bread and 'you know how good it smelled.' She took some on Friday and gained two pounds on Saturday. Starches such as you get in bread are fattening."

The dieters sang Copeland's praises at first, with one woman saying she could pick up a glove that had fallen to the floor without calling for help and another saying she could finally bend down to lace her shoes. Yet the results a few months later were disappointing. Just thirty-five out of the fifty women stayed with the program for the monthlong period of the contest. Four months later, *The New York Times* reported, when Copeland inspected twenty of those thirty-five women, "they were still fat."

"'How many have gained in weight since the class closed?' Six hands were raised. 'How many have lost weight?' Up went eight hands but three wavered and went down." Even the contest winner, Sarah Strong, whose weight dropped from 281 to 250 pounds during the monthlong period of publicly dieting and exercising, "has put on some weight," the paper reported.

They were not the only ones to start out with great hopes and enthusiasm and then fail to lose as much weight as they expected, or to keep it off. It was not just high-protein diets that failed people, it seemed. Low-calorie diets also were not a panacea. Even public figures like Herbert Hoover, who once announced that a low-calorie diet was the answer to his obesity woes, failed to maintain his weight loss. In 1918, he was Fletcherizing and counting calories. A decade later, he was fat again and turning to yet another diet, emphasizing fruits and vegetables and strictly limiting fatty, starchy, and sugary foods, and proclaiming again that it was the answer.

The twentieth century became the age of a diet glut. By the first quarter of the century, all the weight loss basics and diet schemes that are familiar today had been discovered, and promoted. High-protein diets. Behavior modification, in the form of slow eating and excessive chewing. Calorie-counting. Exercise. Metabolic rates. And weight loss entrepreneurs had tried everything from selling reducing belts or thyroid pills, to advising that people eat soap or drink vinegar, to instructing the overweight that they must massage off their fat.

Over the years, those diet schemes were simply recycled, with minor variations. Diets became stricter and stricter, with doctors, around 1928, recommending eating just 600 to 750 calories a day to cure severe obesity. Even that austere prescription was not enough, apparently, and by 1938 the advice was to eat as few as 400 calories a day. The trend reached its nadir in 1977 with a new diet that said you should not even bother to keep your calorie count low. Just eat nothing at all.

That was the advice in a bestselling book, *The Last Chance Diet*, by Robert Linn, an osteopath. To lose weight, he said, you should abstain from all food, surviving instead on a 300-calorie drink called Prolinn that he invented and sold. In Washington, D.C., where Linn opened an office in 1977, politicians and socialites bragged about their weight loss on the Last Chance Diet. Barbara Eagleton, a senator's wife, said she would phone hosts of dinner parties and explain that while she would attend the parties, she would not be eating. That, Eagleton said, is not as bad as it sounds: "It is much easier to sit at a dinner party and eat nothing than just a little bit." The no-calorie diet craze ended a year later, when dieters started to die of heart arrhythmias attributed to a lack of potassium in the diet.

All along there were the strange diets, like Carmen Pirollo's water-cooler diets, that were discovered early in the century and periodically soared to popularity, often remaining in the background, simmering along with a few adherents even when most dieters had moved on to other weight loss schemes. There was, for example, the grapefruit diet, known in the 1920s and 1930s as the Hollywood Diet. It emerged again and again over the years, each time emphasizing few calories, grapefruit, and little else.

Special diet drinks also came and went—one made with skim milk and bananas in the 1930s returned "every decade since in new cans, new flavors, under new names," Hillel Schwartz, author of *Never Satisfied: A Cultural History of Diets, Fantasies, and Fat*, notes. In the 1950s, Rockefeller University scientists devised a low-calorie drink that they gave to obese patients they were studying—the "fabulous formula," *Ladies' Home Journal* called it—which became Metrecal. It was followed by Carnation Slender and, more recently, by Slim-Fast. Did it work? Jules Hirsch, the lead researcher at Rockefeller, said he had given the formula to fat people who had agreed to live at the hospital so that the researchers could study their fat cells. In return, the researchers had promised that they would make the patients thin. Living in the hospital, with no food other than the "fabulous formula" that the researchers provided, they did, indeed, get thin. Then, Hirsch says, they left the hospital to go back to their lives, delighted with their new weights. The weight so arduously lost came right back.

But that, of course, has not kept that general idea—consuming a diet food or diet drink instead of meals—off the market.

"We keep coming back to the same kinds of diets recycled under different names," Schwartz says, "but with different explanations of why they are effective."

Even obesity surgery dates back to the early twentieth century. On November 11, 1911, Dr. W. Wayne Babcock of Samaritan Hospital in Philadelphia reported that he had sliced 12 pounds of fat from a woman's abdomen. He declared that the operation was not risky if the surgeon was skilled. In 1922, Dr. Max Thorek of Chicago, the founder of the American College of Surgeons, reported that his "adipectomies," the surgical removal of fat, required "artistic genius" for cosmetic success.

Now, of course, there is intestinal bypass surgery. Does it work? That depends on what you mean by "work." Most people who have the operation lose large amounts of weight, but their body mass index remains above 30, the criterion for obesity.

By midcentury, America put its own unique stamp on its diet movement. Dieting, the struggle to control your weight, was no longer a solitary pursuit. It became part of the self-help movement, with group support sessions and diet clubs where members encouraged each other, and with leaders, like those of Alcoholics Anonymous, who were reformed transgressors.

The first of these diet clubs was TOPS, for "Take Off Pounds Sensibly," founded in 1948 by Esther Manz of Milwaukee, Wisconsin. Others followed—such as Overeaters Anonymous in 1960, a group modeled after Alcoholics Anonymous and founded by two women in Hollywood. Like alcoholics who had to confess they were powerless over alcohol and ask a higher power for help, so overeaters had to make a similar confession. Of course, overeaters could not exactly swear off food the way alcoholics swore off alcohol. But they had their own version of forswearing food. Instead of eating spontaneously, they were to eat "three measured meals a day with nothing in between."

The next year, Weight Watchers was founded by Jean Nidetch of Queens, New York. Jenny Craig, founded in Australia in 1983, reached the United States in 1985. Those two behemoths grew, dominating all other commercial weight loss programs in the United States. Jenny Craig attracted the Carmen Pirollos who could not abide weighing and measuring food. Weight Watchers, with its magazine, its food products, its Web site, and its medical advisors, gained a reputation for teaching lifelong habits of diet success.

Before long, almost everyone who struggled with weight had either been a member of or seriously considered joining one of the two groups. And for those who wanted something more, there were the programs at university medical centers. As Weight Watchers and Jenny Craig became fixtures in the diet world, university medical centers began offering pretty much the same thing, but with their own imprimatur, the prestige of academe. What they offered, though, was not so different. People would come to group meetings, they would weigh in, they would get a diet or, in some cases, prepackaged diet foods, and they would be taught how to modify their behavior.

All along, diets were accompanied by diet aids, some ineffective, others risky. People tried everything, from thyroid pills in the early years of the century to laxatives, the drug of choice in the 1950s; to amphetamines, which were prescribed with abandon until the 1970s, when they were deemed controlled substances; to phen-fen in the 1990s, removed from the market over concerns that it could lead to heart-valve injuries; to ephedra, removed from the market in 2004, when the Food and Drug Administration determined it could raise blood pressure and lead to strokes and deaths.

Diet books proliferated, some named after their promoters, like *Dr. Stillman's Diet* and *Dr. Atkins' Diet Revolution*. Some diets had names that sounded scientific, like the Zone Diet and the Metabolic Typing Diet, while others bore evocative names of places where the rich and thin hang out, like the Beverly Hills Diet, the Scarsdale Diet, and the South Beach Diet.

As the years went by, the bar for an ideal body got lower and lower. People in the early years of the twentieth century who were thought to be astonishingly slender would never meet the standards set today. Renowned female beauties were becoming skinnier and skinnier. Men were not supposed to have any loose fat—no love handles, no paunches. Yet, at the same time, Americans generally got fatter and fatter, starting in the 1980s and continuing into the new millennium. It seemed that the harder people tried, the more they failed to meet the standards for health and, more important to many, for beauty.

And that, of course, gives rise to the question, Are people struggling because the goals, the ideal body weights, have become unrealistic, or are they struggling because the perfect diet just has not been discovered?

ONE MONTH

It's one month since the diets began, and everyone in the Penn groups, it seems, is losing weight. Even those who cheated have dropped pounds. If one diet is better than another, that difference has not appeared yet. Maybe both are perfect weight loss plans.

"I was a very bad boy this week, and this is the most weight that I've lost," one man in the Atkins group says. "How is that possible?" His transgressions, though, seem pretty trivial to the outsider—they include, he says with chagrin, half a bagel one morning. But their importance, their psychological meaning, was that his iron control was slipping. He had been bad.

An older man says that he, for one, did great and was loving the diet. His weight loss is deserved, well earned. "In some respects my appetite is actually decreasing," he states.

Then a particularly heavy man chimes in, saying he, too, is gaining virtue and with it, its rewards. He had not even lost weight until the past week, but finally, the pounds were coming off. "I went from two fried eggs and two sausages to one egg and one sausage. I went from 10 ounces of steak to 6 ounces of steak. So I'm hopeful," he says.

A young man boasts of his self-control: "I went to the Phillies stadium and got a pork sandwich. I ate it with two spoons, like chopsticks. I just ate the pork and cheese."

As for Carmen Pirollo, he announces that he has been getting the exercise that was urged upon the dieters—he averaged 240 minutes of walking a week, he says—and is sticking with the low-carbohydrate diet plan. "I went to a movie, and everyone is sitting there eating," he says. But he had come prepared, with a special low-carbohydrate snack sold by the Atkins company—"the crunchy type," he explains. He boasts that he has simply lost his craving for the forbidden foods. Even smelling warm, buttery popcorn did not tempt him, he says.

Around the table, his fellow dieters look askance.

"I guarantee you that if you made chocolate chip cookies at home, you'd have two or three or four," one of the men informs him.

Carmen says his doctor, too, had his doubts. "He told me, 'In four months I want to see you, and you'd better lose weight.' He's one of those doctors who is very skeptical about low-carbohydrate diets." His doctor, Carmen says, was happy that he was starting to lose weight. "But he wasn't patting me on the back," Carmen adds.

But the topic for the night is not weight loss. It is thoughts and images that make you want to eat.

"I still have a little bit of a problem when I cook," one man says.

"I have to exert my willpower in the supermarket," says the young man. "I bought a thing of cashew nuts, and pretty soon I was eating them all." Temptation stalked him, he says. "My friend had all of us over for the Flyers game on Saturday. They had four pizzas. It smelled great, and I thought about the positive side of losing weight and what that would do for me." He knew, he said, that if he started eating pizza, if he even took one bite of a slice, all of his resolve would go. "It's like being an alcoholic. That's how I've gotten off the diet before. I have one breakdown and I say, 'That's it.'"

Carmen says he keeps thinking about his goal. "I'm envisioning what I'll look like in July or September. Everyone will say, 'Oh my God.'"

The woman in the group says she thinks about how it would look if she failed to lose weight: "I've told so many people that I'd be embarrassed if I did really badly."

Okay, says Leslie Womble, it is one thing to understand what makes you want to go off the diet program. But can you also point to problem situations and find solutions?

The woman says she had a problem. "I went with my husband's family for dim sum, and everyone ordered communally. I could have ordered for myself, but then it draws all that attention. A lot of the food is wrapped in flour, and the food that isn't wrapped in flour is wrapped in stuff that you don't even know what's in it. You eat little bits at a time. You can't even remember what you've eaten or how much."

Well, says the man who'd been having trouble with his portions of eggs, sausages, and steak, there is a solution, drastic though it may seem.

"Thirty years ago in Massachusetts we went to dinner at Anthony's Pier 4," he says, and when he sat down, he spotted a well-known actress, Angie Dickinson, seated nearby. She was slender, of course, and he sneaked glances at her table to watch what she ate. He can see it still. There she was, elegant, poised, sitting with her friends. Their meals arrived, but the waiter did not bring any food to the beautiful actress. She was not about to eat a restaurant meal: "She brought one bag of carrots and celery, and that was what she was eating."

"So," observes the young man, "one brainstormy idea is to bring your own food."

The woman with the dim sum problem replies she'd thought about that, but she simply could not bring herself to tote her own food to the restaurant. Of course, she adds, she could also have ordered a special meal for herself, but she was chagrined at the thought.

"When I looked at all the food, I thought that there was some that wouldn't be too bad. But if I had ordered the chicken with broccoli, I would look like the odd man out."

There are other ideas, but she rejects them too, thinking she could not have gone through with them. "I thought about eating beforehand and then not eating anything at the restaurant. I could have picked at the food like skinny people do."

Well, says the young man, there is another solution. "Announce to that table, 'I am in this study. I can't have carbs.'" He adds that he's done that. "Everyone I've told has been totally impressed, like, 'Wow, that's so cool.' Not one person has put me down."

Leslie Womble moves the group on to the next talking point, the final lesson for the evening. She wants them to think about what they're going to be discussing when they meet again.

"Next time," she says, "we'll talk about high-risk situations. Let's say you're at the Krispy Kreme. Your wife decides she's going to get a dozen. Does that happen?"

"It happened this week," says a man who finds those doughnuts to be his nemesis.

"The second link is, you buy a dozen," Leslie says. "Every time you get to another link in the chain, your risk gets higher.

"Now let's say you buy the doughnuts and, driving home in the car, you eat a doughnut. Then you put the box of doughnuts on the counter in the kitchen. They are just sitting there. You go to bed. The next day the doughnuts are still there. You see them. You eat one. Then you eat the rest.

"A chain is only as strong as its weakest link. If you see it, break it right away."

3

Oh, to Be as Thin as Jennifer Aniston (or Brad Pitt)

Nearly every woman in America thinks she's too fat, or so women say in surveys by the National Center for Health Statistics. When asked, "Would you like to weigh less?" more than 71 percent say they would.

"I call that question a no-brainer," says Katherine Flegal, a statistician at the National Center for Health Statistics and one of the nation's leading skeptics of the notion that being overweight is necessarily bad for your health. Yet even she is susceptible to the thinner-is-better idea. "What woman *doesn't* want to lose weight?" Flegal asks.

The questions are, How much weight loss is enough? and How thin should a woman be? If movie stars are the ideal, the answers are "A lot of weight" and "Very thin." Jennifer Aniston, for example, reportedly is 5 feet 5 inches tall and weighs 110 pounds. That gives her a body mass index, a measure of weight for height, of 18.3. And it makes her officially underweight and so thin that less than 3.5 percent of American women in her age range, twenty-five to forty-four, meet that standard. Less than 3.7 percent of all adult American women, aged eighteen and over, are that thin.

But if Miss America is the model, even Jennifer Aniston is too fat.

"The perfect Miss America is supposedly 5'8" and 110 pounds," said a Miss America consultant, Samantha Miller, on an Internet site.

Miller reported that she was Miss Virginia in 1997 and knew firsthand the sort of dieting and training that was required to meet the beauty ideal. That year, she said, she collapsed and was hospitalized after she'd stopped eating in her attempt to get thin enough. "At one point I had a problem with anorexia because of dancing and pageants," she says. She is 5 feet 2 inches tall, and her goal was to weigh 95 pounds. "There was intense pressure to lose the weight."

The Miss America pageant has stopped publishing contestants' height and weight. But when one nutritionist, Benjamin Caballero, director of the Center for Human Nutrition at Johns Hopkins University's Bloomberg School of Public Health, examined the pageant's published data from 1922 until 1999, he noticed a pronounced trend. As the years went by, Miss America winners grew taller—their heights increased by 2 percent—but, in a reversal of what you might expect with increasing heights, the women grew ever lighter. The winners' weights actually fell by 12 percent.

In the 1920s, contest winners had body mass indexes that ranged from 20 to 25, slender but well within the range that is deemed a healthy weight. A healthy weight, neither overweight nor underweight, is defined by the federal government as a body mass index of 18.5 to 24.9. A woman who is 5 feet 5 inches tall, like Jennifer Aniston, and weighs 120 pounds has a body mass index of 20. More recently, some Miss America winners have had body mass indexes as low as 16.9. For that, a 5-foot 5-inch woman would have to weigh 101½ pounds.

Yet even though Americans have been getting fatter and fatter, there are quite a few that are, by the healthy-weight standards, just fine. Nearly half—49.5 percent of American women aged eighteen and older—have a body mass index that is deemed "normal," neither underweight nor in the dread overweight zone or the abhorred obese sector.

Why, then, does almost every woman yearn to be thinner? Maybe it's what one anthropologist, George Armelagos, at Emory University, calls the King Henry the Eighth and Oprah Winfrey effect.

In the sixteenth century, when King Henry the Eighth ruled Tudor England, food was scarce and only the rich could afford to indulge themselves. A paunch was a sign of affluence, and the fashion, for men and women, was to be decidedly plump. Now food is cheap in the United States, in England, and in other developed countries. People can get as fat as their bodies allow them to be. But getting thin, thinner than is comfortable, thinner even than is healthy, but thin enough to look like a fashion or beauty icon, takes money. Oprah shows what's involved, with her personal chef, nutritionist, and personal trainer employed to enable her to lose weight. Even so, she struggles and her weight goes up and down.

Men, too, worry about their weight these days, but fashion for them is not quite so brutal, and the result shows in their body mass indexes. National statistics show that men, who can be so judgmental about how women look, are actually the fatter sex—or, at least, the sex with the higher body mass index. Just 36 percent of men over eighteen are at a healthy weight, and a mere 0.9 percent are underweight. The more relaxed male standard for fatness is seen in Brad Pitt, Jennifer Aniston's former husband and a model for male attractiveness. He reportedly is 6 feet tall and weighs 159 pounds. That gives him a body mass index of 21.6, healthy according to federal standards. If Brad Pitt had the same body mass as Jennifer Aniston, 18.3, he would weigh only 135 pounds.

Yet if about half of all American men and women have a so-called healthy weight, whether they like their weight or not, that leaves the other half with an unhealthy weight, according to federal statistics. And one in five Americans is fat enough to be deemed obese. For them, and, especially, for the superfat—the people that doctors call morbidly obese—today's fashionable bodies all too often are a cause for despair. The obese and the morbidly obese, of course, do not look anything like those thin ideals, not even close. And many have never in their entire lives been thin enough to pass for normal. Fat often creeps up on them in infancy, or in toddlerhood, and it never goes away, no matter how hard they try, no matter what diet they go on.

Life as a fat person can be hard, and society's judgment harsh. Studies have found that fat people are less likely to be admitted to elite colleges, are less likely to be hired for a job, make less money when they are hired, and are less likely to be promoted. One study found that businessmen sacrifice $1,000 in salary for every pound they are overweight. Fat people tell researchers that they are accosted on the street by strangers who admonish them to lose weight. Often, their own children are ashamed of them. Studies have shown that even many doctors find fat people disgusting, and some refuse to treat them.

The discrimination starts early. Even children dislike fat children. According to Yale University's Rudd Center for Food Policy and Obesity, directed by Kelly Brownell, the man who developed the LEARN weight loss program, "children as young as three years old associate overweight children with the characteristics of being mean, stupid, ugly, unhappy, lazy, and having few friends. Overweight and obese children are frequently targets of weight-related teasing, jokes, and derogatory names. Peers are common perpetrators of harmful comments, and very often school is the most frequent venue where stigma occurs."

The stories fat people tell are legion.

Tina Hedberg of Conover, Wisconsin, saw a doctor in the summer of 2005, when a diet she was on was no longer eliciting dramatic weekly weight loss. The doctor, she says, told her she had a mental problem because she weighed 400 pounds. She was trying to commit suicide by getting so fat, the doctor informed her. Then the doctor told Hedberg that she had two choices. She could be admitted to a mental institution or, the doctor said, "I could wire your jaws shut so tight that you can't move your jaws to talk, and if you can't talk you can't eat."

Hedberg said that every time she sees a doctor, she is told that anything that is wrong with her is because she is so fat. One time she went to a doctor because her knee was swollen after a fall. "The doctor told me the reason I fell was because I was fat," she says. "He told me there was nothing he could do for me unless I lose some weight."

Miriam Berg, president of the Council on Size and Weight Discrimination, says the same thing happens to her. "Every condition I know of, I have been told the reason for it is that I am fat and need to lose weight to fix it. Including a sore throat. The doctor said I had too much fat around my neck."

She also tells the story of one member of her group, a fat man who happened to be hospitalized when a man in the bed next to him began having a massive heart attack. Doctors rushed in and put paddles on the fat man's chest, jolting him with an electric shock to restart his heart, while the man whose heart had stopped was ignored. "They assumed that if someone was having a heart attack, it had to be the fat one," she said. "So they failed to save the man who was having a heart attack."

In one now-classic study, Colleen Rand, an obesity researcher at the University of Florida, asked forty-seven formerly fat men and women whether they would rather be obese again or have some other disability. Every one of them said they would rather be deaf or have dyslexia, diabetes, bad acne, or heart disease than be obese again. Ninety-one percent said they would rather have a leg amputated. Eighty-nine percent would rather be blind. One said, "When you're blind, people want to help you. No one wants to help you when you're fat."

In another study, Rand questioned 50 women and 7 men who had had bariatric surgery, a weight loss procedure that limits the amount of food that can be eaten or absorbed. All had lost weight. Before surgery, they said, they were embarrassed by their appearance and they faced constant prejudice and discrimination. For example, 77 percent said that their children had asked them not to attend school functions.

Esther Rothblum, a professor of women's studies at San Diego State University, once surveyed fat men and women who were members of the National Association to Advance Fat Acceptance. More than 40 percent of the men and 60 percent of the women said they had not been hired for a job because of their weight. More than 30 percent of her fat respondents said they had been denied promotions or raises because of their weight. One person wrote, "I was told by upper management that I would never be promoted until I lost weight, and the union took management's side."

The respondents told of humiliation. Ninety percent of the fat men and women said that friends or relatives had ridiculed them or made nasty comments to them about their weight, and three-quarters of them said they had been laughed at or derided by fellow employees. One of the survey participants wrote, "While attending a lecture in college, a professor stopped speaking in the middle of a sentence and said, 'When are you going to lose weight? You are really fat.' There were over 100 people in the class."

A quarter of the fat men and 16 percent of the fat women reported being hit or threatened because of their weight. A third said

world wanted to know. Where did Gibson find such a charismatic woman? She came from his own imagination, Gibson replied. She was
his conception, his idea of the great American beauty. "From hundreds, thousands, tens of thousands, I formed my idea. In starting
out in life, each man worthwhile has his ideal of womanhood. A
poet may, perhaps, create his wholly from his fancy. I guess I'm not
a poet. I got mine from the crowd."

The public could not get enough of her, and soon Gibson was
commanding unheard-of fees for sketches of the elusive, ineffably
desirable young woman. In 1903, *Collier's* magazine paid Gibson
$100,000, a sum that would be more than $2 million today, for one
hundred Gibson Girl drawings. Magazines like *Life* sold copies of
Gibson Girl drawings, and women, buying them by mail order, hung
them in their bedrooms. Gibson insisted that the phenomenon had
taken him by surprise. "Now, curious as it may seem, I never consciously set to work to create a special type of the American girl,"
he told *The New York Times* in 1905.

For women who wanted to look like the Gibson Girl, however,
more than just a pompadour and a raised chin were required. The
Gibson Girl was slim, at least compared with prevailing models of
beauty from the nineteenth century, and she helped spur a craze for
ever more assiduous weight loss.

Upper-class women and less wealthy women who nonetheless
strived to look like they were to the manner born wanted to be wil-
lowy, like a Gibson Girl. They were joined by a whole new group of
women who were drawn into the fashion's wake. These were the actresses and chorus girls, the dance hall performers, once so admired
for their voluptuous beauty. With their curvy bodies, their cinched
waists and round hips, their breasts that fairly spilled out of their
bodices, they had cultivated a look of sensual abandon, the look of
women who relished both food and men. That changed with the
start of the twentieth century, when, seemingly overnight, there was
no such thing as a woman who was gorgeous yet heavy. Even actresses like Lillian Russell, one of the great beauties of the nineteenth century, now were derided as much too fat. In 1896, when
reviewers began describing Russell as an elephant, she took up dieting and exercise.

Within fifteen years, conceptions of beauty had changed so much that it was almost inconceivable that anyone had ever found those hourglass-shaped women who pulled their corsets tight so incredibly attractive. "Any girl that looks back and sees what her mothers and aunts looked like at 18 has a moral duty to look different," declared a young man in 1921. As for the beauty of Lillian Russell, it quickly became something for the history books. In 1912, reports historian Lois Banner, the daughter of an actress noticed a photograph in a theater. "'Who is that fat lady?' she asked. The actors present stared at her in shocked amazement. 'Why baby,' her mother said in a low, shocked voice, 'that's Lillian Russell.'"

Men, too, were feeling an increasing pressure to be thin. Within a few years of creating the Gibson Girl, Charles Gibson added another creation, the Gibson Man, a tall, slim companion who immediately set a male fashion standard with his athletic stance and his clean-shaven face. But there were other models for men, too—cowboys, athletes, and so-called dudes, young men who showed up in society columns and who were, notes Banner, "tall, broad-shouldered, and known for their athletic ability."

Meanwhile, fat men lost their stature and their appeal.

They used to be jolly; they used to exude affluence, with their round bellies and watch chains, their vests and their cigars. Many affected a proud bearing and boasted of their weight and the amount of food they could eat. They had their own clubs, the Fat Men's Club of Connecticut, the Heavyweights of the State of New York, the Fat Men's Association. Now the clubs were shuttered; fat men were ridiculed, disdained. "Nobody loves a fat man," actor Fatty Arbuckle famously proclaimed in a 1907 play, *The Round Up*.

Of course, fat men had long been the butt of cruel jokes, and some, like William Banting, plaintively testified that their lives as fat men were a misery, but now the situation was worse, much worse. Now fat was not tolerated in anyone. Now no one, not even the president of the United States, was exempt from the sly remarks.

People laughed when President William Howard Taft got stuck in his bathtub. They gossiped about how the 6-foot 2-inch president, who weighed 275 pounds in 1900, went to Japan, where, notes historian Hillel Schwartz, "an entire village turned out to push him uphill in his rickshaw." One day, Chauncey Depew, a senator from New York, "patted Taft's stomach and asked, 'What are you going to name it when it comes, Mr. President?'" In desperation, Taft brought in a doctor from London to help him lose weight. But his was an all too familiar tale of dieting. At first he succeeded and proudly wore new clothes to show off his newly slim body, but before long he gained back all he had lost.

The problem was that the standards for slimness kept growing stricter and stricter, leaving more and more people behind, unable to meet the new beauty requirements. By the 1920s, women no longer wanted to be Gibson Girls. Now they wanted to look like the rail-thin flappers they saw in drawings by artist John Held, Jr. Like the images of the Gibson Girl, these were *drawings*—and not even drawings of real women. They were drawings of a man's fantasy of women. But they set standards for what a woman's body should look like.

The alluring flapper pictures were appearing on the covers of popular magazines like *Vanity Fair*, *Cosmopolitan*, *Liberty*, and *Smart Set*, but most often on the cover of *Life*. And to show off the flapper body, dresses were short, clingy, revealing. Women with curves were most definitely out of style. "As had been the case with the Gibson Girl, her style—hair, dress, stockings, makeup, jewelry— was marketed aggressively by national advertisers, and young women in cities and towns across the United States dressed and acted in imitation of this new media image," writes historian Carolyn Kitch.

Kitch describes the flapper in Held's drawings as "a tall, thin, cartoonish young woman preoccupied with dancing, drinking, and necking." The flapper, she noted, "was, most of all, vertical," defined by "height and no width," a girl who was "flat-chested and skinny." Held's flapper became the look of the moment. (Kitch also explains the origin of the word "flapper." It came, she says, from a British expression for a young adolescent girl who was still awkward and clumsy, who "flapped.")

And as beauty ideals moved from the slender Gibson Girl to the even thinner flapper, Americans obtained three enabling technologies that are absolutely necessary for most people to live their lives with the nagging worry that they are not thin enough and for some to make dieting their obsession. Without these technologies, the diet industry could never succeed. With them, there were no limits.

The first of these technologies was the bathroom scale, something so common that you would be an oddity today if you did not have one. The popularity of the home scale led to a nation where nearly everyone knows his or her weight to within five pounds, although many people have no idea of such things as their blood pressure, their cholesterol levels, or even their body mass index, which is calculated from your height and weight and is the preferred method today of deciding whether you are too fat.

Incredibly, the bathroom scale did not exist before the twentieth century, and this was not because no one knew how to make one. Instead, companies had not realized there would be such a demand. Until the 1850s, the only scales around were balance scales, used to weigh produce, or grain, or machinery. If you really wanted to know your weight, you would go to a store or a farm, or you would venture into a factory, to step onto one of them.

But with the invention of the platform scale in the middle of the nineteenth century, it became somewhat easier to know your weight. Platform scales began showing up at county fairs, where a barker would guess your weight. Still, regular weighing was unusual. Most people, even if they wanted to be thinner, did not bother with scales, gauging their fatness by how their clothes fit or how they thought they looked.

That changed when the insurance industry began insisting on knowing the weight of people it insured—insurance statisticians had linked high weight with an excess risk of death. By the end of the nineteenth century, the companies were publishing tables of ideal weights and scale makers had discovered a new market—they could sell scales that would weigh people.

At first, companies did not quite get the point, or the psychology, of weight obsession. They made scales that were pretty much the same as the platform scales they were selling to factories and farms, and marketed these unwieldy devices to doctors, who would keep them in their offices, and to grocery stores and drugstores, where you could weigh yourself. The scale makers did not seem to have considered the idea of privacy. You would step onto a metal platform and your weight would be displayed for all to see, on a big round dial. Sometimes the scale would even play loud music or ring when you stepped on it. Gradually, the scale makers figured it out—many people want to keep their weight to themselves—and they began selling scales that allowed a bit more discretion. The music or chimes were silenced, and the person's weight would appear in a little peephole, or on a small printed card.

Around 1900, the first bathroom scales appeared, designed for use in the privacy of the home. They started out as heavy, expensive devices, but as demand grew, manufacturers started selling smaller, cheaper, more attractive scales, and began advertising that weighing yourself daily was essential to health. Before long, weighing yourself, knowing your weight, became almost an obligation. With your own scale, in your own bathroom, you could weigh yourself without clothing and as often as you wished.

The ads for scales showed the new compulsion to keep track of body weight, notes historian Hillel Schwartz. "The 19th-century advertisements for platform scales showed beautifully dressed young women on toe-point, floating over the cast iron with nary a glance toward the weight marked on the balance beam. Advertisements for the smaller bathroom scales in the 1920s showed women in towels, slips, girdles or bathrobes bending over toward the dial in provocative balance."

Along with bathroom scales came another way to learn the blunt truth about your body—the full-length mirror. In the nineteenth century, mirrors, known as "looking glasses," were expensive, "a luxury of the rich," says Cornell University historian Joan Jacobs Brumberg. "They were cherished and passed on from one generation to another," she adds. But by the end of the nineteenth century, Sears Roebuck was selling small, handheld mirrors in its catalogue and "the idea of women looking at themselves so closely was part of a new emphasis on self-scrutiny, defined in the twentieth century as a positive piece of modern femininity."

Full-length mirrors began appearing in big department stores around the same time, allowing middle-class and working women to gaze at their entire bodies when they tried on clothes. By the 1920s, full-length mirrors were appearing in private homes, sold, Brumberg says, "as free-standing pieces of furniture or as attachments to bedroom dressers." Some people made their own full-length mirrors by attaching reflective glass to the back of a door in an apartment, she adds.

As scales and mirrors made it easier to keep track of how much you weighed and what you looked like, another advance let you see what might be humanly possible. For the first time, the technology of photography made it feasible for magazines and newspapers to print photos, says historian Jan Todd of the University of Texas at Austin. Instead of seeing drawings, which could be idealized, you could look at photographs of real people, including models and actresses.

One entrepreneur, Bernarr Macfadden, seized the moment, Todd says, publishing photographs of ideal women, which, to his mind, meant women who were slim and athletic, often stage or film celebrities. And women bought his magazines, poring over the photos. By the end of the 1920s, Macfadden's publications, which included true confessions magazines and one called *Beauty and Health: Women's Physical Development*, had a combined circulation greater than those of the magazines of William Randolph Hearst or Henry Luce.

From then on, there was no turning back.

Of course, even in the 1920s, when standards were looser, women were warned about getting fat. "An excess of flesh is to be looked upon as one of the most objectionable of diseases and must be treated as such," warned Sarah Tyson Rorer, who wrote fifty-four cookbooks and a column for the *Ladies' Home Journal*. Beware of insidious weight gain, she said: "The disease of obesity—for it certainly is a disease—creeps on so slowly that the individual becomes thoroughly wedded to the form of life producing it before he realizes his true condition."

And as the years went by, the weight for an ideal body fell lower and lower. People in the early years of the twentieth century who were thought to be astonishingly slender would never meet the standards set today.

The winner of a 1904 contest in New York for "the world's most perfectly formed woman" was Emma Newkirk, of Santa Monica, California. At 5 feet 4½ inches tall and 136 pounds, she would have a body mass index of 23.3, a healthy weight according to the federal government but with a look that would now be considered chubby.

Historian Lois Banner remarks, "It must be made clear that the 1900 model of beauty, by present day standards, continued to be plump." For example, she says, a variety performer named Frankie

Bailey was famous for her legs, touted, Banner writes, as "the most beautiful in the United States. 'Critics, sculptors, and the general public went into ecstasy over her legs,' one press report declared." Yet, Banner observes, "by current standards, Bailey's legs appear as unexceptional, even pudgy and ill proportioned."

The flappers of the 1920s, so slender for their era, look decidedly chunky by current standards. In 1929, President Herbert Hoover thought he was thin at 189 pounds. Today, he would be told to lose some more weight.

Throughout the twentieth century, thinness, greater and greater thinness, ruled. Even Marilyn Monroe, the archetypical voluptuous woman, was actually quite thin, weighing 115 to 120 pounds at a height of 5 feet 5½ inches. That gives her a body mass index of 18.8 to 19.7, a healthy weight but barely so. If she lost 4 pounds, getting to 111, she would be underweight.

Yet Marilyn Monroe was an anomaly, and as the trend toward thinner and thinner bodies continued, the model women soon were not just thin but emaciated. "By the 1960s," writes historian Carolyn Kitch, "the ideal female body was once again that of a preadolescent girl." This time, however, the model was not a drawing of a stick-figure flapper. It was a real young woman, a British model known as Twiggy. She was 5 feet 7 inches tall and reportedly weighed 91 pounds, which gave her an almost unheard-of body mass index of 14.3.

And even if Twiggy now seems extreme, it was not so long ago that Kate Moss, at 5 feet 6 or 5 feet 7 and reportedly weighing 105 pounds, was an ideal.

Most people may not aspire to the extremely low weight of a Kate Moss or even a Jennifer Aniston. But nearly all who worry about their weight have a dream weight, and for many fat people, the dream weight has become the weight at which, they are convinced, they will be their true selves.

Women fantasize about buying clothes without asking themselves that miserable question: Does this make me look fat? Men think of how it would feel to walk into a store and simply stride over to a rack of clothes that would fit them.

It can be hard to forget you are fat in a society that is unforgiving, the Penn dieters say. Carmen Pirollo says he could not even buy jeans.

"I went to Strawbridge's looking for jeans, but there wasn't anything over a size 36. Then I went to Old Navy. There was nothing over a size 38. I kept looking. Nothing was there. They don't sell them. They don't want anyone that size in the building. If your money is coming from teenagers and young adults, you don't want them to walk in and say, 'This is a fat person's store.'" He is constantly aware of his size. "When I go to my closet I say, 'Dark. What's dark? What's dark?'"

Fat people say they long for a day when they are thin enough to enjoy looking at themselves in photographs. At one of the diet meetings, a woman in the Atkins group confesses, to nods of acknowledgment, that she hates being photographed. "I don't want to see what I look like, and I don't want it duplicated for all eternity."

And fat people say they know that they are being judged by friends, relatives, and strangers because they are so far from the body sizes that are held up as ideals. The subject comes up again and again at the diet group meetings.

Jerry Gordon, a music promoter who is in the study's low-calorie group, explains at one of the meetings: "You don't see gargantuan people in corporate America because appearance is so important and so is being one of the guys." Fat people, he adds, "aren't considered one of the guys.

"I don't know any people who are happy in their heaviness. I don't know any."

But, notes Eva Epstein, the young and slender psychology student who is directing the discussion, "in some cultures, being overweight is a sign of health."

"We don't live there," a man shoots back.

TWO MONTHS

Jerry Gordon and Graziella Mann are fast becoming diet buddies. They have a lot in common—they're middle-aged, they're obese, they have a long history of trying to lose weight, and they have a two-year commitment to the low-calorie group in the Penn diet study. Now, two months into the study, they are laughing wryly and joking with each other about a weight loss that, though steady, seems hardly fast enough considering what lies ahead.

What, asks group leader Leslie Womble, are some of the behavior modification tricks that have been working?

Eating more slowly, Graz and Jerry reply.

"I stretched my time to fifteen minutes at the dinner table—that's a long time for me," Graz says. "I talked a lot and that's one thing I don't do." Her mother, she says, is the one who talks at meals. "I eat," Graz adds. But now she is changing her ways. "I paused between bites. I turned the TV off."

Jerry, too, ate more slowly. "I tried that thing where you put the fork down between every bite. That was really an excellent suggestion. What happened is that it took so damn long to eat the meal that by the end I don't know if I was full but I thought it was time to end the damn thing already."

"It was not like the old days," he adds, "where I would say, 'Gee, where did that 8 ounces of fish go?' or, even worse, 'Where did my dessert go?'"

Graz and Jerry yearned to be in the Atkins group when they signed up for the diet study, and both had the same reason. It was that promise that Atkins makes—you can eat as much as you want as long as you keep your carbohydrates down. And both had long, sad experiences with diets that were so stingy with food that they could not be sustained.

When the diet study began, Graz was at a point in her life when she was ready, more than ready, to get thin and was ready to try almost anything, as long as it was at the University of Pennsylvania. That university, with its weight loss center, was going to supply the diet magic for her. A study there, with the Penn research scientists, was not going to be like those diets she'd been off and on for most of her life.

Graz, dark-haired, with warm brown eyes and a wide smile, remembers well those initial interviews for the Penn study, and she remembers when the investigators gave her a preview of the Atkins diet. Atkins "was the quote unquote in thing," she says, and the diet seemed fine to her. "I said, 'Okay, I can do that.' The line was, you can eat as much as you want. That was the line that caught my attention. That was so appealing."

But when she was assigned to the low-calorie diet, she swallowed her disappointment and thought about her goals.

Graz's mother has diabetes and has to inject herself with insulin, and Graz, who lives with her mother and sees firsthand what her life is like, does not want that. At 223 pounds when the study began, she knew she was at risk. She also, of course, wanted to look good. Her broad grin and friendly demeanor can take her only so far. She wants people to look at her and not think "fat," and she wants to look at herself in the mirror and take pride in what she sees.

"I was always a fat kid," Graz says. "I look at pictures of my Italian family, and they all look like me—short and round. Even my sister, who was always so skinny and so tall. We thought she would never gain weight. She always looked like the perfect lady. Now she looks like me."

Graz tried diets, of course, starting, she says, with "self-made diets" when she was in college: "They would always fail." Then she went to Weight Watchers but found it frustrating. She would sit in the back of the room with the heavier women who were just not dropping in weight, listening while everyone applauded the thinner women who were reaching their goals. "The girls in the back, they're not losing weight. We get left behind."

She and her sister tried amphetamines and lost a lot of weight but "got deathly ill." They tried the Atkins diet, losing weight again, and again becoming ill. "My mother said, 'You're not going to continue.' Being an Italian family, food is major."

Then, two years ago, Graz was in church when a woman came in, wearing a red dress. Graz knew her—she was a mother of five, the youngest of whom was seventeen, and she had always been fat. Now she was not.

"She told me she had been in a program at Penn." So Graz decided that was what she had to do. "Since then, I was waiting to see if the program had come back." Graz works at the university, as a technician in a sleep lab, and so it was easy for her to keep a close watch for announcements of new studies that might be starting and recruiting patients. The announcements, however, always seemed to exclude her. "Every time I saw a program, I didn't have the qualifications. I was too old. I was going through menopause." Finally, the study comparing the Atkins diet with a low-calorie one came up, and Graz seized the opportunity, applying immediately.

She says she knows why she overeats. It is to deal with stress, and maybe also so she will not have to deal with unwanted attention from men.

"There is a lot of stress in my life, and I kept waiting for life to get better. Now I realize that stress will always be there," Graz says. "I had a friend who said, 'The only reason you stayed fat is that you don't want the guys coming after you.' I think there is a part of that, too."

Now she says, "This is my last opportunity to go for it, to go ahead and do it. I am going to forget about things that could go wrong. Life is like that." It is time to commit to being thin.

And the woman in the red dress?

She dropped from sight until the week before the new study began. Then Graz spotted her.

"She was there, at another church. Stupid me. I ran up to her, so excited about my program. It didn't occur to me until I opened my eyes and realized that she was really heavy. I had been waiting to see her. I thought this would be so exciting. That was sort of a downer."

But that is not going to happen to Graz, she has decided. When she loses the weight this time, it will stay off.

Jerry Gordon, who lives in nearby Villanova, Pennsylvania, was fifty-two when the study began and had hoped to join with a friend so they could support each other. His friend had suggested they both sign up. "He wasn't fat enough to make it, but I was," Jerry says.

He, too, had been drawn to the promise of eating his fill on the Atkins diet. "It seemed like it would be much easier. I saw myself going into a Japanese restaurant and eating all the sashimi you want." He also kept noticing people who had lost weight on low-carbohydrate diets. "There's someone who works at the post office who is one of the few people I know who is fatter than me. Now they're shedding pounds," on a low-carbohydrate diet, Jerry says.

Jerry has always struggled with his weight and has tried diet after diet, losing some weight and then gaining it all back, and more. This time, he says, he has a newfound determination to succeed. His blood pressure is starting to climb. He weighs 227 pounds, "pretty overweight," he says, since he is just 5 feet 4 inches tall. And he's the heaviest he's ever been. "I suddenly realized I was in a new phase of my life when you're not as resilient," he says. His goal is to reach 160 pounds. "But any weight loss would be a success," he adds.

4

A Voice in the Wilderness

The problem with Mickey Stunkard—or Albert J. Stunkard, M.D., as his name appears on his long list of publications—is that few want to hear the truths he's discovered about obesity, and many scientists, weight-control specialists, and dieters quickly manage to forget his discoveries as soon as it is convenient. Yet he's a renowned researcher, a grand old man of the field. He started the Center for Weight and Eating Disorders at the University of Pennsylvania—the program that is now conducting the study of Atkins versus low-calorie diets—and he remains its emeritus director. He's professor emeritus of psychiatry at the university and a member of the august Institute of Medicine of the National Academy of Sciences. And his more than four hundred papers appeared in the most prestigious medical journals. But those unpleasant truths he keeps discovering and reporting in those papers somehow just get pasted over with the same old comforting nostrums.

Stunkard stumbled into obesity research by accident, but as it turned out, he was the perfect person to probe long-standing convictions about why some people get fat and why they stay that way. He himself had no personal interest in losing weight—he's tall and naturally skinny, someone who really can eat whatever he wants. He had nothing to prove and was guided only by his curiosity. And he had no particular reason to be suspicious about obesity dogma. In fact, Stunkard had bought into many of the beliefs he ended up demolishing.

His long odyssey began in the late 1940s, when he was still in medical school and planning to be a Freudian psychiatrist, treating common neuroses and psychoses with talk therapy. Obesity and its treatment was the farthest thing from his mind. Until, that is, he met a teenager named Maxine Watters.

Stunkard, completing his training in psychoanalysis at the University of Pennsylvania, was seeing patients who came to the university clinic seeking psychoanalysis. One day, Maxine timidly crept in for her first session. She was a sad adolescent, and that showed in every aspect of her demeanor. Her multitude of problems began with depression and thoughts of suicide. Perhaps not surprisingly, she had no friends. Then she had trouble dealing with her father, who would quietly steal money from his company and make his daughters beg the neighbors for loans so he could secretly pay the money back. And she had a difficult relationship with her obese mother, who spent days behind the closed doors of her bedroom, crying. But the most noticeable thing about Maxine was her weight—220 pounds and going up.

She told Stunkard her problem. "I know that I'm eating too much but I just say to myself, 'What's the use?' and go on eating."

The solution was supposed to be psychoanalysis, so Stunkard began the talk therapy, and at first he thought it was going well. Maxine started to lose some weight and even made a friend at school. But before long, she stopped coming, explaining to Stunkard in a letter that her father told her she could not see Stunkard anymore because she was probably coming to have sex with him.

Ordinarily, that would be the end of the story. Maxine was lost to follow-up, as medical experts say, and Stunkard would simply go on to the next patient. But he and the other psychiatrists in training were trying something new. Tape recorders had just come into use, and they had started taping their sessions with their patients and then meeting as a group to listen to the tapes and discuss them. Stunkard played his tape of his last session with Maxine, hoping that his colleagues could suggest a way to bring her back for more therapy. He says,

> Little advice was forthcoming, and none that brought Maxine back to treatment. But then a remarkable thing happened. We had been listening to the tape of the last treatment session

when suddenly one of our group, a young, obese woman, gasped for air, rose from the floor where we had been sitting, and staggered out of the room. I followed her to find her in the throes of a classic anxiety attack. Reluctantly, she returned to the group and tried to explain what had happened. "It wasn't anything about the father. That was nothing. It was how that girl talked about the way she eats. She isn't hungry in the morning, all morning. Then what it's like at night, how she can't seem to stop eating. Supper doesn't satisfy her, and she just goes on and on. She even gets up out of bed to eat. That's how I eat and I never heard about it before in my whole life!"

Stunkard was stunned and shaken, uncertain what to make of the incident. Then, shortly afterward, another fat patient came in for psychoanalysis, Hyman Cohen, "a huge burly man" aged thirty-seven, a high school teacher. His problem, he told Stunkard, was that he had gained 50 pounds in the last year and simply could not stop eating. "This eating has become an obsession with me," Cohen said. "It's the first thing I think about in the morning and the last thing I think about when I go to bed at night."

Stunkard thought that Cohen had a naïve trust in the power of psychotherapy, but nonetheless began treating him, seeing him in his office for the usual fifty-minute sessions. At first, therapy seemed to be working. Cohen said he had wrested control of his eating, and he lost 20 pounds in three months. Then it all fell apart.

Stunkard tells the story: "One day Mr. Cohen slunk into the office, quiet and subdued. When he stepped on the scales, we could see that he had gained seven pounds during the previous week. He sat silently for a time and then, taking a deep breath, said, 'Well, I have to begin sometime,'" and launched into a tale that shocked Stunkard, a man who had never experienced out-of-control eating and had never heard anything like the episode his patient related.

Cohen's binge began when he cashed his paycheck. "I don't know what happened," he said. "All of my good intentions just seemed to fade away. I just said, what the hell, and what I did was an absolute sin."

He went into a grocery store and bought a cake, pies, and a bag of cookies. Then, Stunkard says, he drove through heavy midtown New York traffic with one hand, pulling food out of the bag with the other and eating it as fast as he could. When he had finished, he set out on a furtive round of restaurants, staying only a short time in each and eating only a moderate amount, in constant dread of discovery. He was not at all sure what "sin" he felt he was committing. He knew only that it was very unpleasant. "I didn't enjoy it at all. It just happened. And when it happened there was nothing except the food and me, all alone." After the restaurants, he bought more cookies and drove home, "with my gut aching from all that I had eaten." He continued to overeat until his next appointment.

Another failure of psychoanalysis, Stunkard thought. Clearly, all that talk therapy had not done much for poor Cohen. The field was fast losing its appeal for him. Patients were not getting better, and he did not feel particularly capable of helping them. "I was very very dissatisfied. I thought I had failed. I just couldn't get ahold of psychoanalytic theory. It didn't help me to understand my patients, and its ideas seemed unconnected to each other and not referring to things I could relate to."

He also was in despair over his own failure as a patient in psychoanalysis. To be trained as a psychoanalyst, Stunkard had to go into analysis himself, but those required sessions were not helping him. "I kept feeling worse all the time. I had entered it to help relieve the anxiety which had troubled me for years. But the anxiety got worse, and after more than two years, I stopped, worse off than when I had started. I was in the depths of despair at having failed as a psychoanalyst and as a psychoanalytic patient."

Then, he said, "in the midst of this turmoil, I remembered a fascinating lecture in medical school. It had been given by Dr. Harold Wolff, a neurology professor at Cornell's medical school in New York, and it dealt with a man named Tom."

Tom had seared a hole in his stomach when he gulped down some boiling hot clam chowder and had ended up with a permanent opening through the muscle and viscera of his abdomen and into his stomach. You could literally look inside, peer into the hole and watch as food entered his stomach, see the food digested, look at the warm wet stomach lining. Wolff befriended Tom and enlisted him as a research subject, persuading the man to allow him to observe how the gastric mucosa changed with emotions.

That, Stunkard decided, was the sort of research he wanted to do, and he wanted to do it under the tutelage of Wolff. He made an appointment to see Wolff, approaching him with trepidation.

"I went to see him and said, 'I was very impressed with your lecture a few years ago when I was in medical school,'" Stunkard recalls. From there, he and Wolff launched into a discussion of Wolff's work, after which Stunkard hesitantly asked whether it might be possible for him to work in Wolff's program. But he needed to find a research project that was compelling enough to hold his attention. So he decided to get some advice from a colleague of his from medical school, Theodore Van Itallie, who was then at the Harvard School of Public Health, working on obesity.

"I called and asked if he thought that obesity might be a reasonable disorder to work on," Stunkard recalls. "Yes, he thought that was a fine idea, and particularly right now." He and his august colleague, Harvard nutritionist Jean Mayer, he told Stunkard, had just discovered the cause of obesity. Their work, Van Itallie confessed, was in rats, but, he explained, it would be wonderful to prove it in humans. The project would be straightforward, he insisted, and he instructed Stunkard on how to proceed.

The idea was that rats eat when their level of glucose utilization falls. That sends a message to the brain that cells are not getting the glucose they need to function. The brain responds by sending signals that make a rat feel hungry, and so it starts to eat. The same effect probably occurs in humans, Mayer and Van Itallie postulated. And when people grow obese, it must be that there is an abnormality that makes it seem as if cells are not getting enough glucose, even when there is plenty of glucose in the blood. People with that abnormality would feel hungry all the time. They would overeat. They would grow fat. So there it was—a simple biochemical explanation of the vexing problem of obesity.

Van Itallie gave Stunkard some advice: "I suggest you take one year and show it works in normal people, a second year to show it does not work in the obese. Then I will make a suggestion you are not going to like. Take a third year. You may take a third year to wrap it all up."

Stunkard was convinced, and approached Wolff.

"I said, 'What would you think if I work on obesity?' He said, 'Splendid idea, work on obesity.'" So Stunkard began what Van Itallie had promised would be no more than a three-year project. The three years stretched out to a lifetime. Needless to say, that simple theory of obesity did not hold up. It turned out, in fact, not even to be true in rats.

But now that he had plunged into obesity research, Stunkard could not bring himself to leave. Question after question seemed to demand a skeptical, rigorous approach, and assumption after assumption seemed to cry out for challenge. He had studied psychiatry, he was trained as a psychiatrist, and he had psychoanalyzed patients. So he was particularly curious about the mental states and the behavior of fat people. Are there psychological reasons that explain why people gain weight or fail to lose it?

One popular notion, advanced in the 1950s by psychiatrist Hilda Bruch, said that obese people got that way because of their parents, in particular their overbearing mothers. Mothers taught children to associate food with comfort by plying them with food as a substitute for affection. It was "the overindulgent and possessive attitude of the mother" that was particularly to blame for obesity, she insisted. Those childhood eating patterns led to a destructive syndrome—children would grow up with a psychiatric abnormality, an "obese personality," as it became known. They would use food as a form of self-medication to soothe themselves or relieve stress.

But was it true? Bruch presented little objective evidence. Yet nearly everyone, including Stunkard, believed that fat people were fat because they were emotionally disturbed. Fat people had psychiatric problems, and their psychiatric problems had caused their obesity.

"There were all sorts of ideas as to how emotional disturbances caused obesity," Stunkard recalled. "The one that sticks in my mind was 'insatiable oral urges.'"

So, in 1961, Stunkard set out to test the hypothesis that fat people are emotionally disturbed. He began with a small pilot study, recruiting eighteen men who were fat and eighteen men who were not.

Issuing a battery of psychiatric tests, he fully expected to find psychiatric traits that distinguished the fat from the thin. But he found nothing. The fat men, he said, "did not differ from a control group of non-obese men, either in the extent of emotional disturbances or in psychological traits—even in 'insatiable oral drives.'"

Still, he thought, even if obese people had no distinct psychiatric disease, perhaps they were more neurotic than people of normal weight. Maybe neuroticism made them fat. As he wondered how to get the sort of data to answer the question, an opportunity presented itself. He was attending a medical meeting one spring in Atlantic City, sitting in a bar and having a drink after a long day of listening to researchers lecture about their data. By chance, one of those researchers, Leo Srole, a sociologist and professor at Cornell University's Medical College, came in, and Stunkard struck up a conversation with him. Just a few hours earlier, Srole had presented his data from a pathbreaking research project called the Midtown Manhattan Study. It was, Stunkard says, "at that time the most ambitious survey of mental illness yet undertaken. It was based on interviews with a continuous sample of 1,660 persons who had been carefully selected to represent a population of more than 100,000." Srole's results had been stunning—20 percent of the group had symptoms of neurosis or psychiatric illnesses, manifested as impaired relationships and impaired performance at work and personal distress. No one had previously found such a high incidence of psychological problems in a community, but Srole insisted his data were telling the truth. Stunkard recalled Srole's statement: "With 1,660 subjects, you really can count on definitive results." And that gave him an idea.

"The mention of large numbers and definitive results intrigued me. I could hardly wait to ask, 'Were your obese subjects more neurotic than your non-obese ones?'

"He paused for a long time," Stunkard recalls. "'You know,' Srole began slowly, 'We never did look at obesity.'"

Stunkard asked him if he had the heights and weights of his subjects. He did. That was all Stunkard needed. With heights and weights, he could learn who was obese and who was not. And with the psychiatric tests, he could tell whether the fat people were more neurotic than those whose weight was normal. Srole agreed to collaborate—he and Stunkard would delve into the data and ask this question.

But the results were puzzling. Obese people were slightly more neurotic, but, Stunkard says, "the problem was that they weren't much more neurotic. The statistical significance was a result of the large sample size; from a practical view, the findings were trivial."

The investigators wrote a paper describing what they had found, although, Stunkard says, they were not sure what, if anything, the results meant. And when they submitted their paper to two journals, both rejected it.

"It seemed a shame that such fine data should come to such a sorry end, and the study kept bothering me," Stunkard said. There must be some meaning to the data, he thought, but he could not figure out how to extract it. Finally, one day when he was in New York's Pennsylvania Station, eating a dish of ice cream and waiting for a train to Philadelphia, he had an inspiration.

"In a kind of reverie, I found myself thinking about the relationship between social class and mental illness. The Midtown Study had been designed to find out if there was such a relationship, and it had found it. So, since we had data on social class, we had entered it into our analyses along with a host of other variables, without thinking about it. I seemed to remember that it had been useful, and if that were the case, it must mean that there was a relationship between social class and obesity. But I couldn't for the life of me remember whether we had found one or not. Then it occurred to me that I had never heard of a relationship between social class and obesity. Had we stumbled upon one?

"I could hardly wait to get back to Philadelphia to look at the data. When I did, the results were stunning—there was a very strong relationship between social class and obesity."

In fact, the data from the Midtown Study indicated that the richer a woman was, the thinner she was. The incidence of obesity was 30 percent among lower-class women, 15 percent among middle-class women, and 5 percent among women of the upper class. One out of every three poor women was obese, but just one in twenty rich women was.

That was the impetus for a barrage of studies asking about the relationship between social class and obesity, and more than three hundred published papers documenting, over and over again, that poor people, and poor women in particular, were more likely to be fat. But it still is not clear why richer women are thinner. Maybe being fat drags you down into poverty—you may get low-wage jobs, or fail to find a husband who makes much money. Or maybe being rich puts social pressure on you to get thin and stay that way. Or maybe being rich lets you pay for programs like weight loss spas and personal trainers and for foods like fresh fruits and vegetables. Some studies have found that fat women are less likely to go to college, that they end up with lower-paying jobs, and that they are likely to marry men of a lower social class, which would argue that being fat leads to downward social mobility. But many obesity experts also point out that people who are poor have less time and fewer resources to pursue weight control and that stores in poor neighborhoods have fewer foods like fresh fruits and vegetables, which are mainstays of many thin people's diets.

There also is a persistent notion that the psychological problems of poverty lead to obesity. But that idea has not been borne out by the data. Stunkard looked for, but never was able to find, evidence that psychological problems were creating obesity. The data in study after study were consistent—obese people had no unique psychiatric abnormalities. Some had problems, such as anxiety, depression, and mood disorders, but in every instance the psychiatric problems were just as prevalent in people of normal weight.

"Most obese people are no different than non-obese people," Stunkard says. They are not eating because they are depressed or because they have a pathological relationship to food or to their parents. If all you had was their scores on psychological tests—if you could not actually *see* the people you were testing—you would not be able to decide who was fat and who was not.

Maybe the obese eat differently, gulping their food or skipping breakfast only to binge later in the day? But no, that also turned out not to be true. Some overweight people eat quickly, some slowly. Some binge, some do not. Some eat when they are stressed; some lose their appetites in those circumstances. And, in every case, thin people are just as likely as the obese to exhibit those behaviors. There is no behavior that is typical of the obese.

The conclusion reached by Stunkard and others who were doing similar experiments was unmistakable: There *is* no psychiatric pathology that spells obesity. And there is no response to food that is not shared by people who are not fat. You can't say you got fat because you, unlike thin people, are unable to resist temptation. Both fat and thin people are tempted by the sweet smell of brownies or the sight of a dish of creamy cold ice cream. You can't say you got fat because there is a lot of stress in your life. Thin people are just as likely to eat under stress. You can't say it was because you used food as a reward. If that is the reason, then why do thin people, who also use food as a reward, stay thin?

Because no particular psychiatric disorder is linked to obesity, the *Diagnostic and Statistical Manual of Mental Disorders*, the American Psychiatric Association's official roster of psychiatric illnesses, does not list obesity. The only eating disorders included are anorexia and bulimia.

No one really wants to hear that, of course. If you are not overeating because you are under stress or because you are sad or because you are celebrating and your mother taught you to associate food with rewards, then why *are* you eating so much? And if there is no behavior that spells doom to your weight-control plans, then what are you supposed to do if you want to stay thin?

Yet, some argue, there are some tiny subgroups of obese people who have psychiatric disorders that lead them to be fat. Stunkard himself is convinced there are two of them. He does not claim that these two disorders are the cause of much obesity. But, he says, for the small number of people who have them, they are responsible for excess weight. Not everyone agrees with his interpretation—some say these disorders are caused by attempts to diet; they are not disorders that make people get fat. But Stunkard says the syndromes, although uncommon, are real. It was his memories of Maxine Watters, the high school student who ate all night, never feeling sated, and Hyman Cohen, the teacher who could not stop eating, that led him to postulate and investigate the syndromes.

He vividly remembered those two patients as he began to focus on obesity: "I began to ask my obese patients about how they ate." Some ate like Maxine, a pattern he named the "night eating syndrome." He concluded that the disorder is a response to stress, that it runs in families, and that patients respond to the antidepressant sertraline (Zoloft) by reducing their uncontrolled eating at night. This is not a disorder of excess hunger, he says. It is a disorder of satiety. Patients say they cannot stop eating once they get started because they never feel satisfied, they never feel full.

The syndrome is rare, Stunkard says, and is not the out-of-control night eating that plagues so many people who are dieting. He estimates that the condition occurs in just 1.5 percent of the population, and it even occurs in people who are not fat, although it is more common among the obese.

Skeptics wonder if the behavior might be caused by a state of semi-starvation elicited by attempts to diet. It is so easy to get into that vicious cycle: You start out each day with good intentions; you *will* be in control. Then, as the day goes on and your body signals you to eat, your iron will breaks down, and once you get started eating, you find it almost impossible to stop. The next morning, you have no appetite because you ate so much the night before. So you don't eat, and you swear, *This is it*, no more overeating. As the day goes on, you get hungry again and start, once again, to eat and eat and eat. You may eat less if you take an antidepressant, but that should be no surprise. Some obese people lose weight if they take Meridia, an antidepressant marketed for weight loss, and they do not have to have night eating syndrome to eat less with the antidepressant.

The psychiatric profession, in its *Diagnostic and Statistical Manual*, has not recognized the night eating syndrome as a psychiatric illness. Yet many people, hearing the symptoms, have responded with relief and gratitude, saying that by describing the syndrome, Stunkard has described their eating and given them hope that there is a treatment that can work. And it still remains a mystery why many fat people have no appetite in the morning, but can be insatiable at night.

Cohen's story, and similar stories related by other fat people, led Stunkard to propose another psychiatric disorder that can result in obesity. He named the syndrome "binge eating disorder," and it has gained proponents who agree that it is a distinct eating abnormality. To have it, you must binge at least twice a week for six months and you must have at least three of six other symptoms: feeling guilty or depressed about your bingeing, eating rapidly, eating until you feel uncomfortably full, eating when you are not hungry, and eating alone so no one can see how much you consume. Its proponents say it afflicts about 2 percent of people, more than half of whom are obese, and usually occurs in people with other psychiatric illnesses. It also occurs in half the people who have gastric bypass surgery to reduce their weight.

But its status remains murky. It is listed in the psychiatry manual as a "provisional diagnosis" that needs more study to determine whether it is a distinct psychiatric illness.

With binge eating, it is not clear what, if anything, will help. Psychiatrists said fat people were bingeing to self-medicate—the eating would raise brain levels of serotonin, the same as an antidepressant drug.

Not so, Stunkard reported. He and others studied binge eaters: some were fat, some were not, but all said they lost control of themselves and would eat huge—*enormous*—quantities of food. If serotonin is the problem, then you should be able to stop that behavior with antidepressants, which raise serotonin levels. Doctors were prescribing these drugs for bingers; but when Stunkard and others did rigorous studies, giving some bingers the drugs and others placebos, it turned out that the bingeing tends to diminish over time in those taking placebos as well as in those taking the drugs. In 2003, reviewing the published papers on the disorder, he wrote that binge eating "appears to be a reactive disorder that waxes and wanes with clinical attention, or no attention at all."

So binge eating disorder remains in psychiatric limbo.

"If you actually talk with people who have binge eating disorder, it takes over a large part of their lives," said Susan Yanovski, director of the obesity and eating disorders program at the National Institute of Diabetes and Digestive and Kidney Diseases. "They don't want to go out because of it. They feel distressed about it. I think this is distinguishable from the normal, everyday binge eating that so many women go through."

Others, like Christopher Fairburn, a professor of psychiatry at Oxford University, who studied bingeing in the general population, scoff at the very notion that binge eating is a psychiatric disorder. "Outside North America, it's basically a laugh," he said. "No one thinks it's a serious condition. There is no literature on it. There are no meetings." And, he added, "whatever you do, including nothing, the bingeing goes away."

But even if night eating and binge eating are real psychiatric disorders that can cause obesity, they are so rare as to have little effect on obesity incidence. And so, if there is no distinctive fat person's eating behavior, no fat person's psychology, what *does* make fat people fat? And why are some people so much more successful than others in losing their excess weight and keeping it off?

Those questions are not a major topic of discussion in the Penn diet study. Despite the years of rigorous research by Stunkard and others, despite the fact that Stunkard himself works in an office just down the hall from the narrow white room where the diet groups gather, the dieters never meet him. The study has a protocol, and it does not include guest speakers. Every group in each of the three medical centers conducting the study is expected to hear the same information, to have the same sort of behavior modification, and to do the same sort of homework—participants write down what they eat and how much they exercise, and fill out sheets on things like their stress levels and situations where food is tempting. That rigid protocol, that insistence that each group hear and do the same things, is the only way to do a rigorous study. If you start mucking around with the different groups, with one group being told one thing and another being told another, you undermine the data. What if dieters had a visit from Stunkard and then ended up with different weight losses than those who did not hear from him? How would you make sense of the study? Maybe the differences would have occurred anyway, simply by chance, and listening to Stunkard had nothing to do with them. Or maybe it did. Scientists simply cannot allow such doubts and questions to creep into their data and analyses. The art of devising a clinical trial like this one is to make sure that every extraneous variable that you *can* control *is* controlled, and that means, in this case, that every single group hears and discusses the same things.

So, as would be expected by the rules of rigorous science, Mickey Stunkard stays in his office and does his research, never poking his head into the rooms where the groups are meeting. No one invites him to drop by and speak to the Atkins and low-calorie groups; no one stresses the question of whether your behavior makes you fat or whether there is, in fact, a behavior that distinguishes fat people from thin. And nearly every one of the study subjects at those diet group meetings simply assumes that psychological factors are part of people's weight problems. They assume that people, for the most part, bring their weight problems on themselves. And they hope and pray that if they can change their behavior, they can control their weight.

Such assumptions, in fact, are pretty much built into the protocol for the study. They form the basis of the behavior modification aspect of the program, and they are a large part of what Leslie Womble and Eva Epstein are providing in those group meetings. When Kelly Brownell was working on his Ph.D. thesis and developing the weight loss program that became LEARN, the program for the low-calorie dieters, he included behavior modification along with it. And over the years, despite the evidence that there is no fat person's eating behavior, obesity clinics have consistently stressed changing behaviors to lose weight. The Atkins dieters in the study did not get the diet part of the LEARN manual, but they got the behavior modification part.

In a way, this is understandable. Studies at academic weight loss centers, including the one at Penn, have found that if dieters meet regularly and are provided with tools to track and change their behavior toward food and to recognize and defuse risky eating situations, they do better, losing more weight and keeping it off longer, than if they are simply handed a diet and told to try it on their own. That does not necessarily mean, though, that the reason the dieters in those groups do better is that they learn to alter or adjust their behavior. It could also be that the better results arise from the accountability that they feel when they commit themselves to coming, time after time, to a meeting where they will be weighed and where they will talk about their eating and whether it is under control. To answer that question—Is it behavior modification or simply coming to meetings with other dieters that makes the difference?—would require another study in which dieters are randomly assigned to one program or the other. And that study has not been done.

The LEARN manual has a section in its introduction that describes and analyzes common beliefs about why people gain weight. Glands, for example, are one excuse, but "the truth is that most overweight people have no gland problems," Kelly Brownell writes. Metabolism is another. And, yes, some people have a faster metabolism than others, he concedes, but "determining your exact metabolic needs is more costly than it is worth, because you approach weight loss the same way regardless of your metabolism." Sixth on the list is "psychological factors." And the section is honest about the research on psychological factors and overeating:

> Many overweight people have trouble controlling their eating in response to stress, depression, loneliness, anger, and other emotions. Does this mean that being overweight is a symptom of deep psychological distress? If so, the remedy would be to root out the underlying psychological problems in hopes that the symptom of overeating would disappear. This theory rings true intuitively for many people but does not have much support among experts. Many normal people have psychological problems but cope without overeating. In people who undergo intensive psychotherapy, weight problems generally remain after their psychological difficulties have been resolved.

But the program delivers an implicit message that psychological problems can cause obesity, with its behavior modification component and its homework sheets that have the dieters write down "thoughts and feelings" right beside the boxes where they describe every meal they have, every morsel they eat between meals. That's also the message when the manual asks, "Did you eat when you were bored, depressed, anxious, angry or lonely? Other feelings may also be involved, like resentment, hostility, jealousy, or even joy. Seeing a pattern is a sure sign that you may want to develop more adaptive ways to cope with difficult feelings."

Yes, there is a subtle difference between saying there is no psychological problem that is unique to fat people and saying that fat people should learn to deal with situations where they tend to eat more than they had planned. Brownell is advocating the latter. But in their discussions at their group meetings, the Penn dieters did not seem to be making that distinction. They simply failed to question the notion that their psychological idiosyncrasies were what underlay much of their problem in controlling their weight.

"I have a tendency to want to eat more between one and five every day," Graziella Mann says at a meeting a little over a month after the study began. "That's when they come at me with things to do. Stress is a big trigger, and I always associate it with that time of day."

Ron Krauss, a 5-foot 9-inch lawyer in the low-calorie group, said his response to his mother drives him to eat. "This has been an ongoing issue," he tells the group. "My mother is five two and weighs about 105 pounds. For the last fifty years she's been saying she has to lose 5 pounds. 'Obsessive compulsive' would be the proper word. It causes me to eat—it's very painful to be around her. But if I ignore her, that creates all sorts of guilt. I saw her on Mother's Day, and she said, 'I see you've lost some weight. You could lose another fifteen pounds.'"

Then, he says, he has "this reward mentality." He explains his internal conversations with himself. "Particularly when things are very hectic and busy and stressful. It's like, 'Have some of this. It will make you feel better.'"

Jerry Gordon, another dieter in the low-calorie group, says his wife's remarks can trigger a psychological response in him that makes him eat. His wife is a slender yoga teacher who never gains weight. "She says, 'Did you have that fill-in-the-blank after I was done eating for the evening?' I say, 'Yes, I did. What's it to you?' She says, 'I feel for you.' That's what gets me fat in the first place."

THREE MONTHS

Ten percent. Three months into the diet study and that seems to be the magic number. Dieter after dieter has lost 10 percent of their starting weight. The question is, Will that be acceptable if it's all they have lost at the end of two years?

The Penn researchers tell their subjects that they should rejoice if they end up with a 10 percent weight loss. The dieters say they would be devastated if they do no better than that. It may well be that most dieters in research studies are lucky to end up with a 10 percent weight loss, but not them. There may be a bell curve of weight loss with 10 percent in the center, but each and every one of these dieters expects to be at the tail end of that curve, with a much bigger weight loss than 10 percent.

Carmen Pirollo says the diet is easy for him. His 10 percent loss—down 24 pounds from his starting weight of 237—was almost effortless, and his friends are starting to comment. "I didn't realize how good it was until people were telling me," he says. "I lost about 7 inches off my waist. I'm on the last notch of my belt now, all the way to the last one." That old diet magic has kicked in.

For Carmen, this is only the start of what he just knows will be a spectacular and permanent weight loss. He cannot imagine that he'll backslide, although he also knows, from his long experience with diets and dieting, that eventually he will reach that dreaded plateau where his weight does not budge and the only thing to do is to stay with the diet and wait it out, knowing that the day will come

It was a lot of weight in a short time, but, Ron says, in part it was because he was using food to soothe himself: "I know there were periods when I have used foods as mood-altering substances."

Now he has gotten used to counting calories and keeping a diary recording what he eats and when he eats it. "It's annoying and it's tedious, but it has two effects. It sensitizes you to what it is you're eating so you don't eat mindlessly, which was always a big problem for me, especially in the evening. And it is a disincentive to eat when you have to look everything up and find its calories and weigh it and write it down. Sometimes I'd just as soon not eat."

He's come to appreciate the wisdom of the diet program: "This is how I'm going to eat for the rest of my life. The more I do it, the more I'm integrating the whole process into my eating. I am eating three meals a day, and I know what a 600-calorie meal is. I know what various snacks are."

His concern is that the study researchers really do not expect him or the others to lose much weight. Why else, he asks, did they tell the dieters that they would be a success if they lost 10 percent of their weight and kept it off? That is almost a nongoal, Ron says. "It's interesting how the people conducting these studies define success in a way that they know we'll be successful."

And his current weight, 214 pounds on his 5-foot 9-inch frame, is not success to him, Ron says. "I don't see why I can't lose a fair amount more. I was thinking I'd like to get below 180. It seems to me there's no reason I shouldn't weigh what I weighed when I was thirty," a time when he weighed 170 to 175 pounds.

Graziella Mann feels like the odd person out. She fell slightly short of a 10 percent weight loss, and she is starting to have real trouble with the diet and wondering what will happen if her weight loss stalls now and peters out.

"I do like the program," she says, "but I'm not getting the results I expected." She started out, at 5 feet 4 inches tall, weighing 223. Then she got down to 209 pounds, and for weeks she has stayed there. "I'm just hanging in there at 209," she says. "They're saying you really need to count your calories, be sure you count everything. That's true, but how can I live like this? I really can't live like this."

She keeps remembering that just before the diet study began, she was asked, Would you be happy with a 10 percent weight loss? That, Graz says, would be about 20 pounds. "I said, 'Yeah, I would be happy, but it's not what I really want.' But they said they would be happy. They consider that a success in the program. I kept wondering why they asked that, and I somehow knew that 10 percent would come back and bite me. Finally, it's come back and reared its ugly head. I said, 'Well, gee, on one hand I'm a success already. I've almost lost 20 pounds, I'm just 5 pounds away.'"

But, she says, "on the other hand, I personally feel like a failure."

5

A Drive to Eat

During World War II a remarkable experiment began at the University of Minnesota, one that would deeply trouble its researchers and would become a classic in the annals of medicine. The question it asked was disarmingly simple: What would happen if young, healthy men deliberately lost a lot of weight?

The study was directed by the late Ancel Keys, a public health researcher at the University of Minnesota whose many accomplishments included inventing the K ration (the *K* was from his last name) for the army when it asked him to find a lightweight food that was packed with nutrients for paratroopers to carry. He also directed a pathbreaking study, the Seven Countries Study, comparing heart disease and diet among twelve thousand men. It began in 1958 and lasted for decades, and its conclusion—that people who ate lots of unsaturated fats, like olive oil, fared better than those whose diet was heavy in saturated fats, like butter—was the origin of the so-called Mediterranean Diet that is promoted today by many nutritionists.

But Keys's weight loss study was very different from his other research. It involved thirty-six young men, conscientious objectors, who took part in lieu of military service. The men were of normal weight and had been carefully selected from a group of one hundred who had applied to participate. The men Keys chose were the healthiest, both physically and psychologically.

For three months, the men were simply studied and observed. Then they started the diet—eating half as much as they normally ate and exercising, walking 22 miles a week. It was the sort of regimen that obese people often undertake when they try to lose weight, and it worked—the men lost 25 percent of their weight over six months. They spent the next three months re-feeding, as Keys put it, increasing their caloric intake and gaining back the weight they lost. Finally, those who remained—four of the men dropped out along the way— were followed for another nine months, when they were allowed to eat as they pleased.

The results were shocking.

While they were dieting, the men were obsessed with food; they could not stop thinking of food and eating. They licked their plates to get every last morsel. Food became the subject of their conversations and their fantasies. They hoarded food; they *fixated* on it.

Keys wrote: "Those who ate in the common dining room smuggled out bits of food and consumed them on their bunks in a long-drawn-out ritual. Cookbooks, menus, and information bulletins on food production became intensely interesting to many of the men who previously had little or no interest in dietetics or agriculture." The men "often reported that they got a vivid vicarious pleasure from watching other persons eat or from just smelling food."

They struggled over urges: to "gulp their food down ravenously" or "consume it slowly so that the taste and odor of each morsel would be fully appreciated." They poured on salt and spices; they started drinking so much coffee and tea that the researchers finally limited them to nine cups a day. They chewed gum nonstop, with one man chewing forty packs a day.

It got worse.

Some of the men began collecting cooking implements, like coffeepots or hot plates. One man found himself poking around in garbage cans. The men began bingeing.

"Several men were unable to adhere to their diets and reported episodes of binge eating followed by self-reproach. During the eighth week of starvation, one volunteer flagrantly broke the dietary rules, eating several sundaes and malted milks; he even stole some penny candies. He promptly confessed the whole episode, [and] became self-deprecatory."

Keys went on: "While working in a grocery store, another man suffered a complete loss of will power and ate several cookies, a sack of popcorn, and two overripe bananas before he could 'regain control' of himself. He immediately suffered a severe emotional upset, with nausea, and upon returning to the laboratory he vomited. . . . He was self-deprecatory, expressing disgust and self-criticism."

The men, previously so emotionally healthy, suffered bouts of depression, irritability, and mood swings. They lost interest in sex—all they cared about was food.

One man wrote, "I am one of about three or four who still go out with girls. I fell in love with a girl during the control period but I see her only occasionally now. It's almost too much trouble to see her even when she visits me in the lab. It requires effort to hold her hand. Entertainment must be tame. If we see a show, the most interesting part of it is contained in scenes where people are eating."

The men's metabolisms slowed to 40 percent of what they were before the study began. Their body temperatures dropped; their heart rates slowed. It was as though their bodies were doing everything possible to conserve calories.

Even when the dieting ended, and the twelve-week re-feeding period was under way, the men had problems. Normal meals were no longer enough. They would eat a huge meal and say they were still hungry.

One man's meals had as many as 5,000 to 6,000 calories, but he "started 'snacking' an hour after he finished a meal." Some of the men consumed 8,000 to 10,000 calories a day.

Keys describes the scene:

Subject No. 20 stuffs himself until he is bursting at the seams, to the point of being nearly sick and still feels hungry; No. 120 reported that he had to discipline himself to keep from eating so much as to become ill; No. 1 ate until he was uncomfortably full; and subject No. 30 had so little control over the mechanics of "piling it in" that he simply had to stay away from food because he could not find a point of satiation even when he was "full to the gills." . . . "I ate practically all weekend," reported subject No. 26. . . . Subject No. 26 would just as soon have eaten six meals instead of three.

Soon afterward, when men who had been starved as prisoners of war during World War II began describing their ordeals, they spoke of the same almost insane behavior, finding themselves dreaming of food and cooking and recipes. One prisoner, Private First Class Risto Milosevich, wrote of his fellow inmates: "They were very hungry. Food—that's the only thing that interested them. Most of the time, you get GIs together and they start talking about girls and ass and screwing, but the only thing they were doing was taking recipes down. In hindsight, it was comical."

An oddity, perhaps. Observations that were ones for the history books, perhaps.

But, a decade later, those troubling behaviors of starving men began to haunt a young researcher at Rockefeller University. They were, he realized, just what he was seeing in obese people who had lost a lot of weight.

The Rockefeller scientist was Jules Hirsch, a man who, like Mickey Stunkard at Penn, has found himself discovering inconvenient truths about obesity and learning that those truths were all too often ignored or forgotten, perhaps because they simply were not what most people wanted to hear.

But if Mickey Stunkard, with his studies of large populations, with his data analyses, was taking one view of obesity, Jules Hirsch, his iconoclastic counterpart at Rockefeller University in New York, was looking at the obesity problem from the opposite perspective. His focus was on individuals and, especially, very fat people who would do anything—even live for months in a hospital on liquid meals—in order to get thin.

In those days, more than half a century ago, the world of research was a different place than it is today. The tools of molecular biology had not been invented, and some physician researchers, like Hirsch, specialized in a very laborious, painstaking kind of work that required taking just a few patients and studying them in minute detail.

The Rockefeller Institute for Medical Research, as Rockefeller University was then called, was a lavishly funded institution on the banks of the East River on the elite Upper East Side of Manhattan, and it had been established for just such studies. The university even had a gray stone hospital, high on a hill on its verdant campus, where patients would live, free of charge, while they participated in research. Then, as now, the only patients in the hospital were people participating in medical studies. Hirsch came to Rockefeller as a young scientist in 1954, lured by what he describes as "a remarkable institution" that gave young physicians time and resources to study diseases or medical conditions for years, allowing them "the extraordinary opportunity of time to reflect on the nature of the disease."

But the hospital and the style of research were not the only attractions for Hirsch. He also wanted to work with E. H. Ahrens, Jr., known as Pete Ahrens, an eminent scientist at Rockefeller who was one of the icons in the then-popular field of clinical investigation. Ahrens was known for his patience and for having the curiosity to embark on long, meticulous studies looking for individual differences in physiological responses. When Hirsch joined his group, the focus was on finding ways to prevent heart disease.

At that time, the powerful cholesterol-lowering statin drugs had not yet been discovered, and diets with very little animal fat were urged upon heart patients and people whose cholesterol levels were high. Hirsch began the work thinking only of heart disease—obesity was the farthest thing from his mind. He had never considered questioning the idea that anyone can be thin if they really want to. Nor did he wonder about the truth of the prevailing wisdom that said that people who never lose weight, or lose and regain, must have some psychiatric issues, some deep-seated need to be fat. In fact, he did not even have a personal interest in obesity—a medium-sized man with a compact body and a square-shouldered stance, he had never had a weight problem. The relationship between diet and heart disease was going to be his research problem.

"The question was, Are vegetarian diets good for preventing heart disease?" Hirsch explains. To find out, the scientists began by asking whether there was a way, other than asking people to recall their diets, to determine what sort of oil or fat they had been eating. It turned out that there was—the fat in food showed up in the globules of fat that float like bubbles in the body's fat cells. Oddly enough, when it comes to fat, you are what you eat.

Ahrens discovered this strange fact by investigating study subjects who had lived in the Rockefeller University Hospital, existing for months on diets that used corn oil as a source of fat. Their fat cells, it turned out, had increased amounts of linoleic acid, the fatty acid found in corn oil. "If you eat corn oil, your adipose tissue gets corn-oily," Hirsch says. "We used to make a joke that if you eat ham, you turn into the Smithfield man."

There had been an epidemic of heart disease in the twentieth century. Had there been a corresponding change in Americans' diets? Ahrens and Hirsch asked. They looked for studies that described American diets, and data from the U.S. Department of Agriculture, which told what Americans ate. And they acquired samples of fat tissue, obtained at autopsies, and analyzed them. Their conclusions were that the American diet had changed from one that emphasized animal fat, and particularly fat from pork, to one with more corn or vegetable oils. The data did not fit with the dogma—if the source of the diet was so important and if people had switched from lard to corn oil, there should have been less heart disease. Maybe obese people, who were more prone to heart disease, were eating more animal fats. Maybe, in fact, animal fat was helping to make the obese grow fat and stay that way.

But no, the investigators reported. They did not just ask obese people what they ate—they examined fat tissue from obese people. And, they discovered, obese people were eating the same fats as the non-obese. "Therefore, their diets, at least in the kind of fat being consumed, were not a significant factor in the production of obesity," Hirsch remarks.

But once he started looking at fat cells from obese people, Hirsch noticed something peculiar. Those fat cells were huge and numerous, very different from the compact, almost petite, and much less plentiful fat cells of people of normal weight.

That was interesting, he thought. What would happen to fat cells if obese people lost weight? Would there be fewer of them and would they be smaller, or would the formerly fat people keep all their fat cells but deflate the cells down to almost nothing?

It should be a straightforward study. Hirsch decided to advertise for a few obese people who would agree to live at the Rockefeller

University Hospital for eight months, during which time the scientists would control their diets and make them lose weight. Everyone would benefit—Hirsch would get his before-and-after samples of fat cells, and the obese patients would become thin.

Obese people, seeing the ad, eagerly volunteered, and Hirsch recruited four of them, each of whom had been fat since childhood or adolescence. These were not just slightly overweight people. They were fat, truly massive.

One man, C.F., was thirty-eight and weighed 350 pounds. A thirty-six-year-old woman, R.S., weighed 280. A forty-year-old man, C.A., weighed 340 pounds. The fourth patient was E.L., a man who weighed 320 but had weighed more than 400 pounds two years earlier before losing more than 100 pounds on his own.

The study subjects began with an agonizing four weeks of a maintenance diet to assess their metabolism and caloric needs. They lived in the hospital, and their food was limited to what the scientists provided, with diets that were carefully adjusted to keep their weight steady, high as it was. Only then, after Hirsch knew how many calories each of them needed and how quickly each burned calories, could the diet begin. Although no one realized it at the time, that initial maintenance phase would be critically important in understanding what happened to those fat people during and after the study.

The weight loss phase that followed the maintenance phase was difficult—a period of four to five months when the subjects' only nourishment was a liquid formula providing 600 calories a day. Finally, the subjects spent another four weeks on a diet that maintained them at their new weights.

The long ordeal seemed worth it, though. Everyone lost weight, 100 pounds on average. Everyone was delighted with their new, slimmer selves. And everyone, including Hirsch, assumed that the subjects would leave the hospital permanently thinner.

That did not happen. Instead, Hirsch says, "they all regained." He was horrified. What an incredible setback, what a terrible consequence for people who had spent more than half a year living in a hospital and who had endured most of that time subsisting on just 600 calories a day. And they certainly wanted to be thin, so what went wrong? *Why*, Hirsch wondered, did the pounds come back?

He found himself mulling over the problem. Was it that fat tissue grows back, restoring itself when you take it away, much in the way that the liver regenerates when you remove part of it or that skin grows back over a wound? But no, that could not be, Hirsch realized, because he knew of a situation in which surgeons remove a large chunk of fat and it does not regenerate. "I often reflected that people who have large fatty tumors, called lipomas, and had the tumor removed did not regain the weight," he said. That means that a large mass of fat tissue can be removed and the fat never returns. But what happened with dieting could not be the same, he decided. His subjects kept their fat cells, but the cells had lost their fat globules and shriveled in size. "Shrunken adipose tissue over the entire body behaves in a very different way and restores itself," Hirsch observed.

There was, of course, another possibility that could explain the shocking weight gain without evoking some mysterious process in which fat tissue restores itself. Maybe it was just that those four people had some deep-seated psychological need to be fat. Perhaps other fat people would stay thin once they got their weight down.

So Hirsch and his colleagues, including Rudy Leibel, who, at the time, was working with Hirsch at Rockefeller, repeated the experiment and repeated it again. Every time the result was the same. The weight, so painstakingly lost, came right back. But since this was a research study, the scientists looked at more than just weight loss; just as in the first study, they measured metabolic changes and psychiatric conditions and body temperature and pulse. And that led them to a surprising conclusion: Fat people who lose large amounts of weight may look like someone who was never fat, but they are very different. In fact, by every measurement, they seemed like people who were starving.

On every count, the weird, bizarre, almost depraved behavior that Ancel Keys reported when he studied the young men who were deliberately starved in his experiment during World War II was just like what Hirsch observed among the formerly obese subjects at Rockefeller University Hospital. Something was driving those people to regain their weight, and it was not a deep-seated desire to be fat.

Their bodies, for example, had changed so that they hung on to, clung to, every calorie that was eaten, making it harder and harder for them to stay thin. Before the diet began, the fat people had a normal metabolism—the number of calories burned per square meter of body surface was no different than it was for people who were thin and had never been fat. That changed substantially when they lost weight, with the formerly fat people burning as much as 24 percent fewer calories per square meter of their surface area than the calories used by those who were naturally thin.

The Rockefeller subjects also had a psychiatric syndrome that had been termed "semi-starvation neurosis." Hirsch's patients dreamed of food; they fantasized about food or about breaking their diet. They were anxious and depressed—some had thoughts of suicide. They secreted food in their rooms. They daydreamed about food. And they binged, looking for all the world like ordinary dieters who binge, looking like Mickey Stunkard's patient Hyman Cohen, who had told the stunned Stunkard that he had completely lost control of himself.

That story had shaken Stunkard, making him doubt the power of psychotherapy. But Hirsch's study was saying that perhaps there was another explanation. Cohen, like the fat people who had lost weight in the Rockefeller studies, was behaving just like someone who had been starved.

The Rockefeller researchers explained their observations in one of their papers: "Perhaps the most intriguing aspect of this study was that the removal of obesity by means of caloric deprivation led to behavioral alterations similar to those observed in the starvation of non-obese individuals. It is entirely possible that weight reduction, instead of resulting in a normal state for obese patients, results in an abnormal state resembling that of starved non-obese individuals."

Eventually, more than fifty people went through the months-long process of living at the hospital and losing weight, and every one of them had these physical and psychological signs of starvation, Hirsch reports. There were a very few who did not get fat again, but they made staying thin their life's work, becoming Weight Watchers lecturers, for example, and always counting calories and maintaining themselves in a permanent state of semi-starvation.

Did those who stayed thin simply have more willpower? In a funny way, they did, Hirsch says. "The strange thing is that it really

does have to do with willpower in the sense that extremely powerful and very disciplined minds can force the body to accept and maintain a weight-losing or even low-weight-maintaining diet. But there
is a biochemical or basic biological element in what it is that we call
'willpower,'" Hirsch says. "And the dichotomization of mind versus
matter is not a very helpful way to attempt an understanding of obesity. Yet that is exactly what everyone does in and out of the sciences."

Could it be that the problem with obesity is that some people are just
weak-willed at some point in their lives and allow themselves to
gain unconscionable amounts of weight? One way to interpret Hirsch
and Liebel's studies on the near impossibility of permanent weight
loss for the massively obese would be to propose that once you get
fat, your body adjusts, which makes it hopeless to lose weight and
keep it off. Maybe if you let yourself get fat, you seal your fate: being
obese becomes normal for your body. The question was important
because if getting fat was the problem, there might be a solution to
the obesity epidemic—convince people that any weight gain was a
step toward an irreversible condition that they most definitely did
not want to have.

But it turned out that the answer to that question was not what
many had hoped. That uncomfortable discovery began with studies
in Vermont around the same time as Hirsch was doing his studies in
New York and that continued into the 1980s as a few scientists
probed further. The studies were done in different ways by different
researchers and in different populations, but they all found the same
thing. Yet perhaps because their results cast into question everything
that is commonly believed about gaining weight, they have become
known mainly to research scientists and ignored by the general public.

The first experiments were the inspiration of a scientist, Ethan
Sims of the University of Vermont, who asked what would happen
if thin people who had never had a weight problem deliberately got
fat. This was, of course, the reverse of the famous Ancel Keys experiment, but that was not how or why Sims thought of it.

Sims says he got the idea from research he had done during a sab-
batical year, when he was trying to make mice fat. That turned out to

be difficult—even when they were supplied with abundant tasty food, the mice ate only enough to maintain their weight. Sims could force-feed the animals, but then they would increase their metabolic rate and burn more calories, which led them to gain less than was predicted. Even if the animals put on some weight, they would lose it and go right back to their original weights when the study ended. Sims began to wonder whether people, too, would have a hard time gaining weight. No one had ever really asked—who, after all, would want to get fat?

But Sims was a university faculty member, and when he returned to the University of Vermont he managed to find subjects for his weight-gain study among its students. He deliberately recruited students who had never been fat and had no family history of obesity and who were willing to make a serious effort to try to become fat. It sounded as if it would be easy—all you would have to do is indulge yourself with all of your favorite calorie-laden treats. Most people, when asked, say they could weigh much more than they do but that they exert their willpower to keep their weight down.

But Sims and his student volunteers found otherwise. To their own surprise, these subjects found it all but impossible to gain much weight; no matter how much they tried to eat, they just could not become obese. The experiment was a failure. Could it have been that deep down the students really did not want to be fat? Was it really that hard to gain weight?

Maybe, Sims decided, the problem was that the volunteers were free to move about and were burning too many calories with physical activity. He thought of the perfect subjects, people who really would have no chance to cheat and burn off calories: prisoners. So he repeated his experiment with men who were incarcerated in a nearby state prison and who volunteered to become fat.

This time, the experiment worked, in a fashion—the men got fat. But producing obesity turned out to be much harder than Sims had anticipated. The men increased their weight by 20 to 25 percent, but it took four to six months for them to do this, eating as much as they could every day. Some ended up eating 10,000 calories a day, an amount so incredible that it would be hard to believe, were it not for the fact that the research study had attendants present at each meal who dutifully recorded everything the men ate.

But when Sims calculated the amount of weight the men *should* be gaining, he discovered that they were gaining much less than would have been predicted and that different men gained at different rates. Once the men were fat, Sims asked how many calories they needed to maintain their weight and how that compared with the calories they needed when they were at their normal weights, before the study began. The answer was astonishing: When the thin men got fat, their metabolism increased by 50 percent. They needed more than 2,700 calories per square meter of their body surface to stay at their obese weight, but just 1,800 calories per square meter to maintain their normal weight.

Maybe all fat people have very fast metabolisms, strange as that might seem. But no. Obese people who got that way naturally turned out to have perfectly normal metabolic rates, no different from the average metabolic rate of a thin person who is at a weight that feels comfortable and easy to maintain.

Then Sims did another study. He recruited very heavy men and dieted them down to the same level of fatness as the newly obese prisoners. These men, while just as fat as the prisoners, needed half as many calories to maintain their weight. That, of course, was just what Jules Hirsch had found, but the results helped convince Sims that his striking findings with the men who gained weight were correct. The men who lost weight were like the mirror image of the gainers.

As for the fat cells of the newly obese prisoners, it turned out that they had simply grown larger, much larger, but their number remained constant. The men were fat, but they got that way by stuffing the cells they already had with globules of fat, not by growing more fat cells. So, because they always had fewer fat cells than people who were naturally fat, they were fundamentally different from naturally fat people.

When the study ended, the prisoners had no trouble losing weight; within months, they were back to normal and effortlessly stayed there.

The implications were clear. There is a reason that fat people can't stay thin after they diet and that thin people can't stay fat when they force themselves to gain weight. The body's metabolism speeds up or slows down to keep weight within a narrow range. Gain weight and the metabolism can as much as double; lose weight and the metabolism can slow down to half its original speed. That, of course, was contrary to what every scientist had thought, and Sims knew it, as did Jules Hirsch.

In a review article published in 1976, Sims wrote, "Ever since Lavoisier demonstrated animal respiration, there has been a tendency to assume that animals constantly burn their substrates with the same even flame and the same even efficiency." But, he added, "there is no reason to believe that this maximum is achieved or is constant in different individuals under different conditions."

Hirsch wrote his own summary of the work:

The body weight of an obese or nonobese person tends to remain constant. When the system for controlling fat storage is challenged by experimental over- or under-feeding, energy expenditure alters as a counter force, "bucking" the change. The overfed person increases fat storage but burns more calories, which acts as a brake on further accumulation of fat mass. The reverse occurs with weight reduction; a decline in body fat storage leads to a decrease in the burning of calories.

The message never really got out to the nation's dieters, but a few research scientists were intrigued and asked the next question about body weight: What determines whether someone will be fat or thin? Is body weight inherited? Or is obesity more of an inadvertent, almost unconscious response to a society where food is cheap and abundant and oh, so tempting? An extra 100 calories a day will pile on 10 pounds in a year, public health and obesity experts are fond of telling us. Keep it up for five years and you'll be 50 pounds heavier.

Of course, everyone has seen fat families—photos of fat parents with their fat children have become almost a cliché in today's obesity-obsessed nation. And everyone has seen families in which the parents are slender and all their children are thin. But there are two possibilities that could explain why the children of fat parents are fat: it could be that the children inherit a genetic tendency to be fat, or it could be that the parents encouraged bad eating habits and an abhorrence of exercise. Growing up in a household where gargantuan portions are the norm, or where the kitchen is always stocked with tempting chips and nuts, cookies and ice cream, might make anyone fat. Or so it would seem.

That is the assumption behind today's push to change the food offered in schools, getting rid of soda machines and replacing high-fat meals with ones with less fat. It is the assumption behind the movement to ban junk-food advertising that is directed at children. And it is the assumption behind the assertions that people today are fat because there are too few bike paths or sidewalks or because schools are not devoting enough time to physical education. The assumption is that your environment determines your weight.

Mickey Stunkard, ever the iconoclast, wondered if that assumption was true and, if so, to what extent. It was the early 1980s, long before obesity became what one social scientist calls a moral panic, but a time when those questions of nature-versus-nurture were very much on his mind.

Stunkard wanted to study adoptees—a classic method of deciding the relative contributions of genes and environment to human traits. But he needed large numbers of people who had been adopted in infancy and reared apart from their biological parents, and he needed to know the height and weight of the biological parents, the adoptive parents, and the adoptees. Such information is not available in the United States, where adoption records generally are sealed and there is no national database of adoptions. But, by chance, Stunkard discovered what looked like a perfect way to address his questions—it turned out that there was an adoption registry in Denmark that should have all the information he needed.

The registry had been developed to study mental illnesses. It was instituted by Harvard psychiatrist Seymour Kety, who had worked with researchers in Denmark in his quest to understand whether schizophrenia was inherited and had used that country's meticulous medical records of every adoption there between 1927 and 1947, including the names of the adoptees' biological parents. But when Kety used the registry for his research study, the results were disappointing. Schizophrenia was so rare in that Danish population, occurring in just 0.5 percent of the people, that he could not conclusively establish whether a tendency to develop it was inherited or not.

Stunkard, however, saw an opportunity to answer his questions about obesity. One day, when he and Kety were talking about the registry, he popped the question. "I said, 'My goodness, do they have heights and weights [of the people in the registry]?' He said yes, they have heights and weights, but why would that matter?" Stunkard explained that he might be able to use the Danish registry to determine whether body weight is inherited. Kety agreed to write to the Danish psychiatrist Fini Schulzinger, who oversaw the registry, and with that introduction, Stunkard went to Copenhagen to meet with Schulzinger and beg to be allowed to use the data.

The visit was unsuccessful, Stunkard recalls. "Schulzinger said, 'Well, Dr. Stunkard, we are the psychiatric institute. All we deal with are psychiatric issues, and obesity is a somatic issue and we don't deal with that.'"

For five years, Stunkard pleaded with Schulzinger, but got no further. Finally, he gave up. He had learned of another adoption registry, in Iceland, and scientists there seemed eager to allow him to do his study. So he got a plane ticket to Iceland to meet with the geneticists there. It turned out that for the same price, he could continue on to Copenhagen after staying in Iceland. Why not? he thought, and made the arrangements.

"When I arrived in Copenhagen, Schulzinger said, 'I have someone to work with you.' I said, 'On what?' He said, 'On the adoption registry.'" Astonished, never understanding why Schulzinger had suddenly changed his mind, Stunkard leapt at the chance. What he thinks of as his five-year courtship of Schulzinger was over. He could finally get down to answering that nature-nurture question with rigorous and extensive data.

Stunkard's Danish collaborator turned out to be "a very, very young guy," Thorkild I. A. Sorensen, who had never published anything but who was enthusiastic and willing. The researchers did their analysis of the registry data and began writing a paper. "I would write a draft and mail it to him. Two months later, he would send it back to me with his comments," Stunkard says. "I think we spent three years writing that paper. Then we sent it to the *New England Journal of Medicine*. They took it right away."

And no wonder. The study included 540 adults whose average age was forty. They had been adopted when they were very young— 55 percent had been adopted in the first month of life, and 90 percent were adopted in the first year of life—and reared apart from their biological parents. The investigators divided the adoptees into four categories: thin, average weight, overweight, and obese. Then they mailed general health questionnaires to the adoptees' biological parents and their biological siblings, asking for, among other things, their height and weight.

The results, published in 1986, were unequivocal. The adoptees were of the same fatness as their biological parents, and their fatness had no relation to how fat their adoptive parents were.

The scientists summarized their data: "The two major findings of this study were that there was a clear relation between the body-mass index of biologic parents and the weight class of adoptees, suggesting that genetic influences are important determinants of body fatness; and that there was no relation between the body-mass index of adoptive parents and the weight class of adoptees, suggesting that childhood family environment alone has little or no effect."

It did not matter what the children's adoptive parents fed them; it did not matter whether they set a good or a bad example with their diets and exercise habits. The fatness or thinness of children when they grew up had nothing to do with their adoptive parents. It had everything to do with the fatness or thinness of their biological parents, even though the children may have had no contact with their biological parents and may not even have known them.

In their paper, Stunkard and his collaborators pointed out the implications:

> Current efforts to prevent obesity are directed toward all children (and their parents) almost indiscriminately. Yet if family environment alone has no role in obesity, efforts now directed toward persons with little genetic risk of the disorder could be refocused on the smaller number who are more vulnerable. Such persons can already be identified with some assurance: 80 percent of the offspring of two obese parents become obese, as compared with no more than 14 percent of the offspring of two parents of normal weight.

A few years later, Stunkard conducted another study, using another classic method of geneticists—investigating twins. This time, he used the Swedish Twin Registry, which included nearly 25,000 same-sex twins born in Sweden between 1886 and 1958. He looked at 93 pairs of identical twins who were reared apart, 154 pairs of identical twins who were reared together, 218 pairs of fraternal twins who were reared apart, and 208 pairs of fraternal twins who were reared together.

In a paper published in 1990 in the *New England Journal of Medicine*, Stunkard and his colleagues reported that the identical twins had nearly identical body mass indexes, whether they had been reared apart or together. There was more variation in the body mass indexes of the fraternal twins, who, like any siblings, share some, but not all, genes. The researchers conclude in their paper that 70 percent of the variation in people's weights may be accounted for by inheritance, which means that a tendency toward a certain weight is more strongly inherited than nearly any other tendency, including those that favor the development of mental illness, breast cancer, or heart disease.

One of the study's researchers, Jennifer R. Harris of the Karolinska Institute in Stockholm, said in an interview when the study was published that the results mean "almost all of the differences in weight between members of a population are due to genetic differences." Stunkard said the study "confirms with an even more powerful message than before that genetics play a major role in determining body weight."

The results do not mean that people are completely helpless to control their weight, Stunkard says. But they do mean that those who tend to be fat will have to constantly battle their genetic inheritance if they want to reach and maintain a lower weight.

And, as another investigative team discovered, some people will have a much tougher battle than others. That study, by Claude Bouchard, who directs the Pennington Biomedical Research Center at Louisiana State University, and his colleagues, found scientific evidence supporting what almost everyone has noticed—that some people can eat all they want and never gain weight. His paper, published in the same issue of the *New England Journal of Medicine* as Stunkard's paper, provided the first demonstration that different people who overeat by the same amount can gain very different amounts of weight.

Bouchard recruited twelve pairs of identical twins, young men who agreed to purposely try to gain weight. This was not a repeat of Ethan Sims's study, in which he tried to make normal-weight people obese. Instead, Bouchard was asking whether different people, overeating by the same amount, would gain the same amount of weight. By using twins, he could ask whether people with identical genes would gain identical amounts of weight if they overate by the same amount.

So for six days a week, over a period of one hundred days, each young man deliberately ate 1,000 calories a day more than he needed to maintain his weight. The total number of extra calories for each man was 84,000. With 3,600 calories per pound, that meant that each man should gain 23.3 pounds.

The average weight gain, Bouchard reported, was 18 pounds, but the number of pounds gained varied from 9½ to 29 pounds. Identical twins tended to gain nearly identical amounts of weight and tended to put on fat in the same places. One pair would put on weight in the thighs, another in the abdomen, another in the buttocks.

Bouchard also tried to understand why there were such pronounced differences in weight gain, and he noticed something intriguing. Those who gained the least weight converted most of their excess calories to muscle protein, and those who gained the most converted most of their extra calories directly into fat. It takes nine times as much energy to turn food into muscle as it does to turn it into fat, which helps explain why the twins who turned their extra food into muscle burned up most of their extra calories.

"We definitely have some very efficient people who are good at gaining weight," Bouchard said. When the study ended, however, all the young men effortlessly returned to their original weights, just like the subjects in Sims's studies of overfeeding.

Stunkard said the two studies together gave a scientific reason why some people struggle so hard to keep their weight under control. For these people, the data "gives them a nonjudgmental, reasonable explanation. It tells them that genetically, they've got the dice loaded against them." And, Stunkard added, he hoped the studies would persuade people to abandon psychological explanations for obesity that were so popular at the time, like "insatiable oral urges" and "defective impulse control."

They also provided evidence for a phenomenon that scientists like Hirsch and Leibel were certain was true—each person has a comfortable weight range that the body gravitates to. It might span 10 or 20 pounds—someone might be able to weigh anywhere from 120 to 140, for example, without too much effort. That may be why so many people say they could easily gain weight if they just let themselves go; they could, in fact, gain weight, but there is a limit to how much they would gain. Going much above or much below a person's natural weight range is difficult, and the body fights back by increasing or decreasing the appetite, and increasing or decreasing the metabolism to push the weight back to the range it seeks.

"This is not good news," Bouchard says. "Over the past decade we have seen repeated a thousand times studies in which people have lost weight but then regained it."

Jeffrey Friedman, an obesity researcher at Rockefeller, wrote in the journal *Science* about the powerful biological controls over body weight:

> Those who doubt the power of basic drives, however, might note that although one can hold one's breath, this conscious act is soon overcome by the compulsion to breathe. The feeling of hunger is intense and, if not as potent as the drive to breathe, is probably no less powerful than the drive to drink when one is thirsty. This is the feeling the obese must resist after they have lost a significant amount of weight. The power of this drive is illustrated by the fact that, whatever one's motivation, dieting is generally ineffective in achieving significant weight loss over the long term. The greater the weight loss, the greater the hunger, and, sooner or later for most dieters, a primal hunger trumps the conscious desire to be thin.

He added that people often can lose 10 pounds or so, but beyond that it becomes increasingly difficult to lose large amounts of weight and keep it off.

"In trying to lose weight, the obese are fighting a difficult battle. It is a battle against biology, a battle that only the intrepid take on and one in which only a few prevail."

The difficulty, the dieters insist, is that they are so afraid of losing control. It is not just thoughts and images. It is being on a knife-edge, worried that a tiny push will spell doom.

Leslie urges the dieters to plan ahead when they know temptation lurks and to find other things to think about, other things to do—like going outside for a walk—when food is calling to them.

Ron Krauss says that the entire exercise, trying to play little psychological games with yourself so you will not eat, seems futile.

"The fundamental concept is that you are having this dialogue with yourself where one part of you is trying to fool the other part," he says. He elaborates after the session is over:

"Lots of times I'll have a conversation with myself. 'Gee, I really could go for some ice cream.'

"'No, it's not good for you. It's just a short-term thing, a short-term pleasure.'

"Two minutes later, I am going to say to myself, 'I really want some damn ice cream.'" End of conversation.

One man finds the words to ask the unspoken question that underlies all the talk about willpower and keeping temptations out of the house. It is one thing to resist Krispy Kreme doughnuts while you are losing weight, or to tell yourself that celery—*celery*—is a snack. But how, he asks, can you live this way for the rest of your life?

"This is what I don't get about weight loss and dieting," he says. "How do you get the reasons why you want to lose weight to be important enough to maintain that self-control forever?"

It is a paradox, he says. He knows from his own experience that it is possible to refuse food, to be totally uninterested in it, for religious reasons. But not, he fears, for reasons of staying thin.

"We keep a kosher home, and you can put the most delicious-looking lobster and crab cakes on the table and I'm not going to eat them. It's because I don't eat that food." But what happens when he is dieting? he asks. He can try to talk himself out of eating something he wants but should not have, but all too often, as Ron Krauss pointed out, he will eventually just stop the internal dialogue and go get the food he craves. He can try the behavior modification methods the group is being taught, like going for a walk, calling a friend, or getting out of the house, to take his mind off of food, but they do not make much difference. What he wants is that food, and all too often, before the night is over, he eats it.

What, he asks, is going on? He was able to decide to eat only kosher food and never look back. Why can't he decide to eat only foods that are permitted on his diet?

It is not as though he always restricted himself to kosher food. He took up that strict diet seventeen years ago, just after he married, when he made a choice to eat only kosher foods from that day forward. He never had any problem with his decision, and he had no regrets.

"I remember the very last night. We happened to be on a cruise, and I said this is the last time in my life that I won't be eating kosher food. I had lobster and escargot," both of which are forbidden on kosher diets. After that, such food lost its appeal, no matter how hungry he was.

"I had a friend whose mother passed away, and I went to his house. He had catered kosher food, but it wasn't my house. It wasn't my food. I wasn't going to eat that food," he says, because he could not be sure all the kosher rules were followed. "I was able to spend three hours there, and there was never a doubt in my mind that I was not going to eat that food. I didn't even have a glass of water because it was not my glasses."

But, he said, he can't make himself not want snacks that he knows are forbidden on his diet.

"Last night, I was watching TV and I wanted ice cream." He could not resist the urge. The more he tried not to think about it or to tell himself that his goal was to be thin, the more he had to have it. Finally, of course, he went to the freezer and dished it out.

"The only thing I can come up with is that the reasons I want to lose weight—I want to feel better, to look slimmer, to look better—are not powerful enough.

"I want to do it," he says. "I want to lose weight." But maybe, he adds, he does not want it enough.

"I'm looking for that little magic key that makes it easier. And I know that key does exist. If someone said, 'Peanuts aren't kosher,' I would never eat a peanut again. But if someone said, 'Peanuts make you fat,' that isn't enough."

6

Insatiable, Voracious Appetites

So what does make you want to eat? What makes you unable to stop? If nothing else, the annals of medicine reveal that at least for some people, at least in some circumstances, something is going on in the brain that compels them to eat. And whatever that drive is, it can be impossible to consciously control. Wanting to eat less works for only so long. Eventually that drive, powerful as the urge to drink water or even the drive to breathe, takes over.

That was a hard-earned lesson for research scientists, though, and it only emerged after a century of science and a slow, painful, tortuous path of discoveries that began long before the studies with people who agreed to starve themselves or to try to gain weight and that continued for more than a century. It went on haltingly and with great difficulty while scientists like Mickey Stunkard studied twins and adoptees and while one diet guru after another promoted what were claimed to be failure-proof ways to lose weight.

The gradual unraveling of the brain circuits that control eating began with the story of a fat little boy, and came to include rats that were so voracious they ate themselves to death, and mice so grotesquely obese that although they could barely move, they could not stop stuffing themselves with food. It was the work that would finally uncover the secret pathways deep inside the brain that determine how much food is eaten and how much food is enough. And unless those brain circuits were found, researchers knew, dieters would be left forever with that old and not terribly useful advice that dates back to

Hippocrates: To control your weight, simply eat less and exercise more.

The story begins at a time when there were almost no tools to probe the human brain. It was the dawn of the twentieth century when a young boy walked into the office of an Austrian physician, Alfred Froehlich. The first thing you would notice about the boy, referred to in case histories as R.D., was that he was fat.

The child was born in 1887 and was slim until March 1899, when he suddenly began gaining weight. Two years later, when R.D. was fourteen, his despairing parents took him to see Froehlich. The doctor performed a detailed physical exam and, questioning the boy, learned that obesity was just one of his problems. The boy's genitals had not developed, the vision in his left eye was failing, and he complained of excruciating headaches, saying it hurt when Froehlich tapped on his skull. All those symptoms added up to a pituitary tumor, Froehlich reasoned. That meant that the boy's best hope was an operation to remove the growth in that gland in the base of his brain.

Froehlich saw the tumor, a white-sheathed glistening orb, as soon as he opened R.D.'s skull. It was just where he thought it would be. "In the depth of the sphenoid sinus, the whitish membrane of a cyst the size of a hazelnut was encountered. After incision in the midline, several spoonfuls of a fluid resembling old blood drained out. By measuring with the finger and comparison with the roentgenogram [an X-ray-type photograph], it could be ascertained that the cyst which contained the fluid corresponded to the hypophysis [pituitary gland]," Froehlich wrote. He removed the tumor, and "there was considerable improvement in the general condition."

That seemed to indicate that the brain, and specifically the pituitary, might be where the eating-control centers were located, providing evidence that obesity could be a glandular disease. Fat people, or at least some of them, might be lacking in pituitary hormones, whether or not they had actual pituitary tumors. There was no treatment— no drugs to replace pituitary hormones were available. But at least there seemed to be a diagnosis and a medical explanation for obesity.

Before long, doctors were diagnosing "pituitary insufficiency" or "Froehlich's syndrome" in fat child after fat child, especially if the child was a boy with what looked like underdeveloped genitals. Of course, since pudgy boys often have accumulations of fat that partially hide their genitals, doctors were finding it easy to make the Froehlich's syndrome diagnosis, to Froehlich's dismay. He insisted that the condition was extremely rare, "though every little fat boy has been named after me."

It turned out that the pituitary was not quite the right part of the brain to control eating, although it was close to the correct region. Froehlich was misled because R.D.'s pituitary tumor also had compressed brain areas around the pituitary. The true brain center that controlled eating was not discovered until the 1940s, when scientists found a way to selectively destroy small areas of the brain in white rats and learned that if they hit the right spot, they could make animals grow very fat.

The experiment itself was stunning, an amazing demonstration that obesity can originate in damage to a tiny area of the brain and that animals can develop insatiable appetites, even eating themselves to death.

The first paper appeared in the *Anatomical Record* in 1940, written by two scientists at Northwestern University who used an electric current to kill brain cells in the hypothalamus, a small gland, shaped like a cone, at the base of the brain. The hypothalamus directly connects to the pituitary and controls fundamental reactions, like fight or flight, and the regulation of temperature, thirst, and also, these scientists discovered, eating. The procedure, reported the scientists, A. W. Hetherington and S. W. Ranson, was straightforward. First they anesthetized the animals, and then, using electric probes, they made two lesions on each side of the hypothalamus. "The pair of lesions on either side invariably fuses into one large area of damage," they wrote. When the animals woke up from the anesthesia, the scientists watched what happened. As it turned out, the rats began to eat.

This, however, was not normal eating. It was *gorging*. Within months, the rats were enormous, with some weighing twice as much as their littermates, which served as controls.

The animals were packed with fat, stuffed with globs of slick, shiny adipose tissue, Hetherington and Ranson said. Their autopsies revealed that the rats "invariably" had "enormous accumulations of adipose tissue in the abdomen," so much so that "it is sometimes difficult to dissect out the ovaries and adrenals."

Others repeated the experiment, watching with fascination as the animals they operated on became ravenous, and obese. In 1943, three Yale scientists—John Brombeck, Jay Tepperman, and C.N.H. Long—reported that rats in one experiment were eating so greedily that three animals, still groggy from the anesthetic, inhaled food into their lungs, and one actually asphyxiated itself. The rats, the scientists reported, "voraciously gnawed and ate chow pellets before their pharyngeal reflexes were sufficiently re-established to maintain an adequate airway." When they autopsied the rat that died, they saw that its entire digestive system was stuffed like a sausage with rat chow, from its esophagus, to its pharynx, to its stomach.

It was an effect so striking that it became almost legendary, "repeated from teacher to student and colleague to colleague and sometimes slightly embellished in the process," as one report has it:

> As the tale is usually told, the aftermath of the surgery proceeds something like this: As soon as the rats awaken, even before they have shaken off the effects of the anesthesia, they stagger to the trough of rat chow and plunge in, gobbling down pellets as if their lives depend on it and stopping only when their stomachs could hold no more. After enough time has passed that some of the food has made its way into the intestines and created a bit of room in the stomach, the rats began to eat again.

The rats were eating three times as much as normal animals, and when the researchers tried to restrict their food intake by putting just a normal amount of food in their cage, the fat rats avidly gobbled it down, "consuming in some instances a day's portion in less than an hour." The animals were not picky eaters—they devoured anything edible put in their cages.

Like Hetherington and Ranson, the Yale scientists autopsied their animals: "Many of the animals were almost incredibly obese, with an increased amount of fat in every depot of the body." Their livers were so full of fat that those organs weighed twice as much as normal.

Of course, what happens with rats may not reflect brain controls in humans. But there were hints from sporadic reports of brain-injured patients that the hypothalamus played the same role in people. The earliest published report, from 1840, involves a woman who suddenly grew hugely obese before dying at age fifty-seven. On autopsy, doctors saw that a large brain tumor had compressed the entire base of her brain, including the pituitary and the hypothalamus.

Others, over the years, had their own anecdotes of patients who inexplicably grew very fat.

Steven B. Heymsfield, who was the deputy director of the Obesity Research Center at St. Luke's-Roosevelt Hospital in New York, told of a fourteen-year-old boy who was hit by a car when he was sledding and suffered a brain injury involving his hypothalamus. The boy was of normal weight until his accident. Afterward, "he became 400 pounds, literally in weeks."

The rat experiments were almost too tantalizing. They meant that it was possible to create obesity in rats. They showed that there was a region of the brain that controlled eating in rats. And they supported observations that the same region appeared to control eating in humans.

Yet with the discovery came a frustrating problem. Scientists could not figure out what the hypothalamus was doing, or what it was secreting or failing to secrete, that made the animals grow so fat. Nor could they answer the obvious question: Could the experiments with rats help explain, and cure, human obesity?

It took three decades before the next breakthrough came, and this time it involved a different species—mice—and did not involve the destruction of parts of the brain. The first of these mice was discovered by accident in a research laboratory, and appeared born to be fat.

The mouse, like the rats, had a voracious appetite, but it had no obvious brain damage. It was massively obese, so fat that the rats paled in comparison. It was so fat that it could barely move, so fat that it spread out like a round puddle of fur on the floor of its cage.

It was found by a caretaker at the Jackson Laboratory in Bar Harbor, Maine, a research center that collects and maintains mutant strains of mice. Scientists send interesting specimens to the lab, but no one knows where this particular specimen came from. The caretaker saw it one day in 1949, a monstrous mouse sprawled out in a cage. It was barely moving, and it was simply huge.

A graduate student came to take a look, but decided it was nothing more than a mouse that was pregnant. The mouse, however, was not pregnant. It was a male, in fact, and it was one of the fattest animals ever seen, three to four times heavier than a normal mouse. It also ate three times as much as a normal mouse. The mouse was given a designation, *ob* (pronounced "oh-bee"), for "obese," and bred to create a line of fat mice. Yet researchers were stymied when they asked why it had gained so much weight.

So the *ob* mouse languished, an interesting curiosity, but little more than that. Then, sixteen years later, in 1965, another strain of mutant mice turned up at the Jackson Lab, weighing about twice as much as normal mice. This time, though, the animals had an additional problem—type 2 diabetes. The strain of mice, named *db* (pronounced "dee-bee"), for "diabetes," were making enormous amounts of insulin, the hormone made by the pancreas that allows cells to use glucose for energy. Somehow, though, just like people with type 2 diabetes, the mice were not responding to the insulin they made.

Douglas Coleman, a scientist at the Jackson Laboratory, decided to study the *db* mice, not to learn why they were fat but to figure out diabetes. If these mice made huge amounts of insulin, he reasoned, they might also be secreting a chemical signal that tells the body to make insulin. His plan was to find that chemical by isolating it from the animals' blood. But first, he had to assure himself that the *db* mice were making such a chemical, and to do that he decided to physically attach a *db* mouse to a normal mouse, so that blood from one flowed into the body of the other. If the *db* mouse was making something that signaled insulin production, the normal mouse would then start making massive amounts of insulin.

The operation involved slicing one animal open along its right side and another along its left side. Then Coleman cut a small hole in each animal's abdominal membrane. He lined the mice up and sewed them together along the holes in their membranes. Finally, he sewed their bodies together along the cuts made in their skin. The result was two mice attached side by side, like conjoined twins, with their circulations mixing through the hole in their abdominal membrane.

It was an unusual operation, and Coleman, like most scientists, had never tried it. So he blamed himself when his first few conjoined mouse pairs died, assuming that it was because he lacked surgical skills. The mice, from the same genetic strain, were nearly identical twins, so, in theory, there should be no immunological rejection when they were attached.

Then he noticed something very strange. When the mice died, it was the normal mouse that died first. But those normal mice were no longer normal. They were thin, very thin—*emaciated*—with no fat at all on their bodies and no food in their stomachs or intestines. Did they eat? Coleman wondered. He hooked *db* and normal mice together and carefully observed them. The fat mice ate, just as always, but the normal mice behaved like anorexics, or worse. No matter how hard they tried, Coleman and the animal caretaker could never catch the normal mouse sneaking even a nibble of mouse chow. Once the normal mouse was hooked to the fat one, it never ate again, as far as Coleman could see. It simply starved to death.

Coleman had no idea what was happening, but as he searched the medical literature for clues, he noticed a paper from a decade earlier, in 1959, in which scientists had hooked normal rats to fat rats that had had their hypothalamuses destroyed. The same thing happened—the normal rats stopped eating and starved to death. The researcher, G. R. Hervey of the University of Cambridge, suggested an explanation: The fat rat, he proposed, must be making some substance that was supposed to instruct it to stop eating, but it could not respond to the signal. As it got fatter and fatter, its body kept making more and more of the stop-eating substance, but to little avail. But when the fat rat was hooked up to a normal rat, the normal rat suddenly was exposed to a flood of that stop-eating signal in the fat rat's blood. The normal rat responded appropriately. The chemical told it to stop eating, and it did, eventually starving to death.

That explanation, Coleman reasoned, might be the reason why a normal mouse starves to death when it is hooked to a *db* mouse. But then, he wondered, what about the *ob* mice? Would an *ob* mouse hooked to a normal mouse also make the normal mouse die of starvation? And what would happen if you hooked an *ob* mouse to a *db* mouse?

Coleman set off to find out.

The answer was perplexing—the *ob* mice were the opposite of the *db* mice. When he hooked an *ob* mouse to a normal mouse, the normal mouse would be fine; it would eat the same amount as before the operation and would maintain its weight. This time, it was the *ob* mouse that was changed when the two animals were conjoined. When an *ob* mouse was attached to a normal mouse, the *ob* mouse stopped eating, not so much that it starved to death but enough so that it ate less than ever before and became thinner than such mice ever had been.

There was a likely explanation, Coleman decided. Ordinarily, a mouse controls its appetite by making a substance that Coleman thought of as a satiety factor, a chemical that tells its brain it does not need any more food. By making just the right amount of this factor, a normal mouse neither grows fat nor wastes away. It eats just enough to maintain its weight and stops eating when it has had enough.

The problem in *ob* mice, he decided, must be that the animals lack the satiety factor. Without that signal, the animal's brain reacts as though the animal were starving to death, instructing the animal to eat and eat and eat, making the animal monstrously fat. That also meant that if you hooked an *ob* mouse to a normal one, the *ob* mouse would get some of the normal mouse's satiety signal and eat less, growing thinner than it would otherwise be.

The problem in *db* mice, Coleman reasoned, must be that they cannot respond to the satiety factor. The *db* animals would make more and more of the substance, trying to tell their brains that they were fat enough. But, as though their brains were deaf to the signal, the animals would just keep eating and eating.

So, according to Coleman's hypothesis, the difference between an *ob* mouse and a *db* mouse is that the *ob* mouse does not make the satiety factor and a *db* mouse makes it but does not respond to it.

Coleman published his work in 1973, in *Diabetologia*, a journal for endocrinologists, providing the data and his logical explanation of what must be going on.

Of course, it seems irresistible to ask whether such a satiety substance underlies human obesity. Maybe some fat people are like the *ob* mice, unable to make enough of the satiety substance, which is why they grow fat, while others may be like the *db* mice, making plenty of the substance but failing to respond to it. Maybe there are degrees of an ability to make or respond to the substance, which would explain why some people are fat, some are overweight, and others are skinny. It would seem that obesity researchers would immediately jump on the intriguing clues from the mutant mice and start looking for the satiety factor, whatever it was.

But Coleman was working in a different era than today's, when nearly every finding on obesity—even in animals—is publicized. And Coleman was not part of the obesity researchers' clique. Few had heard of him, and those who had often were not convinced that studies of mutant mice had much to do with human obesity. Obesity specialists continued to believe that people overate because they had psychological problems. If you could learn to find other ways to fill the emptiness inside you, or if you could break the habits you learned at your mother's table—to see food as a reward or to always clean your plate—then you could become thin and stay that way. Obesity treatments stressed psychological counseling and behavior modification.

There was evidence to the contrary—Mickey Stunkard, for example, did his studies in the 1960s showing no psychological differences between fat people and those of normal weight. Jules Hirsch was publishing his studies in the late 1960s and early 1970s on obese people who had lost weight at the Rockefeller University Hospital and ended up looking normal but with the physiology of someone who was starving. Ethan Sims, in the 1970s, had published his studies of the prisoners in Vermont who had agreed to gain weight and found it so hard to do so. But the idea that obesity was largely a manifestation of psychological problems prevailed. And even if the mice did hold lessons for humans, it was hard to extend Coleman's seminal work. You would need to find the satiety factor and see whether fat people made less of it or were less responsive to it. But that factor, if it existed at all, was elusive. Coleman himself spent the rest of his career, until his retirement in 1991, looking for it, but to no avail.

Most obesity researchers, if they thought about it at all, would say that Coleman had embarked on a futile quest. "At the time, a lot of people didn't think *ob* mice would be informative," says Jeff Friedman. "People thought it was an inexplicable finding" that the mice grew so fat. Friedman, however, thought that Coleman was onto something, and he made it his mission to complete the task, to find the satiety factor.

Back when he was just starting out in science, Friedman thought that the secret to weight control would be simple. There would be a chemical signal sent from the stomach to the brain, telling the brain that the person had eaten. People who are overweight may not make enough of this chemical, and so the way to help them lose weight would be to supply more of it.

That was the 1970s, when researchers had just discovered a similar brain system that controls the response to morphine. They found that the body makes its own morphine-like substances, which scientists named endorphins, and that endorphins can latch onto brain cells to create a sensation of calm and well-being.

Friedman had worked on the endorphin system as an apprentice in the laboratory of Mary Jean Kreek of Rockefeller University. "I was just dumbstruck and fascinated by the idea that molecules could modulate behavior," Friedman says. "I had imagined human behavior as this metaphysical event. The notion that you could explain this major human behavior by a set of molecules really captivated me."

Eating, he thought, was likely to be controlled in the same way, and he might be able to figure it out. The plan was to isolate and identify the satiety signal. He knew, from Coleman's work, that *ob* mice did not have that chemical telling them to stop eating and that they had a mutation that apparently disabled a gene, the *ob* gene, that controlled production of the signal. No one had isolated the *ob* gene, but scientists had an idea of what it might be. Many thought it directed the synthesis of a protein, cholecystokinin, or CCK, that is produced by the gut after eating. If so, CCK would be the satiety signal. And, in support of this notion, there were reports that CCK signaled mice to stop eating and that its levels were lower in the brains of *ob* mice.

But while some scientists had reported that a dearth of CCK was one reason that *ob* mice grew so fat, one of Friedman's colleagues, Bruce Schneider, had his doubts. In his experiments, it looked as if there was the same amount of CCK in the brains of *ob* mice as in the brains of their normal-weight littermates. One test of whether CCK was the satiety factor that had gone awry in *ob* mice would be to determine where the CCK gene was located. Scientists knew that the *ob* gene was on chromosome 6 in mice. If the CCK gene was actually the *ob* gene, it would have to be on chromosome 6.

There was a scientist at New York University, Peter D'Eustachio, who had studied the chromosomal location of the CCK gene, so Friedman and Schneider sent him a letter. "We said, 'We would like to know what chromosome CCK is on,'" Friedman recalls. "'Is it on chromosome 6?' The answer came back: The data are consistent with it being on chromosomes 4, 9, or 10. But not 6.

"Still, we were hopeful," Friedman says. Maybe D'Eustachio was wrong, or maybe the scientists at the Jackson Lab who had reported that the *ob* gene was on chromosome 6 were wrong. He and Schneider would do one more set of experiments, and this study would answer the question unambiguously. Using a radioactive tracer to monitor CCK production, they would ask whether the *ob* mice made normal amounts of CCK. If CCK was the satiety factor, those fat mice should not be making it.

The answer was clear. Not only could the obese mice make CCK, but they made it in amounts that were indistinguishable from the amounts made by normal mice. Whatever the *ob* gene did, it was not directing cells to make CCK.

"You get a result like that and the question becomes, What in heaven's name is the *ob* gene?" Friedman says. "At some level, the animals have a behavioral mutation. How does a single gene determine such a complex behavior?"

He became obsessed with the gene, determined that he would find it and that it would reveal the brain's secret ways of deciding what is eaten and how much.

He and Schneider already were convinced that people have only limited control over the amount they eat and what they weigh. Both knew the work of Hirsch and Leibel and of Sims, and both accepted it, while realizing that it contradicted the prevailing wisdom about psychological factors. Both Friedman and Schneider had become convinced that body weight is genetically determined, as tightly regulated as height. Free will, when it comes to eating, is an illusion.

"People can exert a level of control over their weight within a 10-, perhaps a 15-pound range," Friedman says. But expecting obese people to decide to simply eat less and exercise more to get their weight below the obesity range, below the overweight range? It seldom happens. Any weight that is lost almost invariably comes right back.

Still, we all can decide to eat or not, choosing to skip dinner, say, or pass up dessert. Isn't that free will? Not really, Friedman says. The control mechanisms for body weight operate over weeks, even years, not day to day or meal to meal.

He knew that there was a body of psychological research asking what determines how much people eat in one sitting, and he knows it continues to this day, an endlessly fascinating exploration of behavior. One of its leaders is at the University of Pennsylvania— psychology professor Paul Rozin.

Rozin likes to devise little experiments to show that you can easily manipulate how much people eat and that social cues can lead people to eat more, or less. You can think you are ready to eat simply because the clock says it is time for a meal. Diet plans often tell you to try to make a small portion seem big. Put your dinner on a salad plate, or pour your breakfast cereal into a small bowl. That can work, Rozin says. But being a scientist, he asks, What are the limits to tricking your eye?

Rozin and his graduate student Andrew Geier tried a little experiment with pretzels. Geier lives in a seven-story apartment building with 180 apartments where, three days a week, sixty big, soft Philadelphia pretzels, a local delicacy, crusted with salt, are put out on a table in the vestibule for the residents. People come by and help themselves and almost always take the same amount—each person takes a single pretzel. For three weeks, Geier hung around at the end of the day, counting how many pretzels were left. The number was nearly constant—twenty.

So Rozin and Geier began slicing the pretzels in half and watching what happened. People would be free to take two halves if they wanted to. But they did not. Many who used to take a whole pretzel instead walked away with half of a pretzel. At the end of the day, sixty halves remained.

What about something smaller? Rozin put Tootsie Rolls in a bowl, leaving them out in the psychology department office, and watched his colleagues. Most took one as they strolled by. He cut the candies in half—most still took one piece, half of a Tootsie Roll. He tried the experiment again with miniature Tootsie Rolls, which are a quarter the size of the regular ones. The results were the same—people took a piece. If he cut them in half, they usually took half as much.

But, Rozin says, this doesn't work with M&M'S. Half an M&M is just too small a portion—people take a handful of the candies, and no one cares if that handful contains halves or whole pieces.

If people take half as much of larger items, the argument that large portion sizes are making people fat gains some support. Maybe people are being led to eat more, a lot more, than they would eat if they were simply served less. Rozin suspects that is happening. He loves to compare the United States and France, a country in which portions are much smaller and where people do not ordinarily snack between meals.

"If you use megasizes," Rozin says, referring to containers that hold much more than normal, people take more. "You pour more Coke from a bigger bottle. It even happens with laundry detergent. If you have a bigger box of Tide, you pour out more."

Brian Wansink, director of the Cornell University Food and Brand Lab, documented the effect. In one experiment, Wansink asked what happens if you give moviegoers a huge tub of popcorn as opposed to a simple box of popcorn. With the tubs, people ate 45 to 50 percent more.

Just having a food like pretzels out in plain sight, easy to reach, makes people eat more, Wansink found. To show this, he put chocolate in offices. If the candy was on a plate, easy to see and easy to reach, people took, on average, nine pieces a day. If the chocolate was kept in a desk drawer, so that you had to deliberately open the drawer to get it, people ate six pieces a day. And if it was kept out of sight and a few yards away from a person's desk, the average was three pieces a day.

But the popcorn and pretzel experiments, the study with Tootsie Rolls, and the one with soda assumed two things. First, big portions of food are making people fat. Second, eating more food at one meal, or in one snack, or at one movie, has no effect on what you eat the rest of the day. You will go on to eat the same portions of the same food later on, taking in more calories than you would if you had had half a pretzel or a smaller tub of popcorn or if you had never gone to that movie at all. Does that happen, or do people compensate over the day, or the week, or the month?

Rozin confesses that researchers have not carefully addressed that question: "It's inconvenient, empirically inconvenient, to study people over a few days. So people do what is easy."

And Friedman's work casts doubt on the popular interpretation of those experiments of Paul Rozin's and Brian Wansink's. Friedman would say that you can't just observe people at one brief time, or even for a day or a week. That is not how the body controls its weight.

"People live in the moment. They lose weight over the short term and say that they have exercised willpower," Friedman says. But he adds, "It appears that over the long term, this basic drive wins out." And just as willpower cannot make fat people thin, a lack of it does not make thin people fat.

Just look at the amount of calories a person consumes, he says. If you eat about 2,000 calories a day, you consume about 730,000 calories in a year. If you try to meticulously count your calories, you will err, because tables of calorie counts are not precise. Inevitably, you will make little mistakes. You'll make a mistake when you try to estimate how much a cube of cheese weighs (cheese is 100 calories per ounce, but is that cube an ounce or is it an ounce and a half?). Or you might not include that handful of raisin bran you tossed into your mouth as you measured out a cup of cereal. You would be lucky if your errors were within 10 percent of your true calorie count.

You inevitably make little errors in trying to count your calories, but there is no way your body can allow such imprecision and keep its weight stable. Body weight tends to stay nearly steady year after year. If your body's control system were off by 10 percent in the number of calories it instructed you to consume, you could be getting 73,000 fewer calories over the course of a year, which translates into a weight loss of 20 pounds, or you could be getting an extra 73,000 calories, a weight gain of 20 pounds. If your body were as imprecise as you are in counting calories, your weight would fluctuate wildly and unpredictably.

Bruce Schneider had not even needed such arguments, or the studies of the *ob* mice, to convince himself that the body exerts a tight control over its weight. The revelation came to him when he was a medical resident with an erratic schedule. Some days he was living at the hospital, sleeping on a cot, eating whatever he could whenever he could, making meals out of candy bars from vending machines. Other days he was off duty, sleeping all morning, going out with friends, eating at restaurants.

"I weighed myself every day, but I had no idea how many calories I consumed or how many calories I burned," Schneider says. But day after day, his weight was rock steady—145 pounds.

Intrigued as he was with the idea of searching for the *ob* gene, in the end Schneider decided that he did not have the heart for it. It was going to be a long and tedious project with no assurance of success even after years and years of work. He moved on to other things. Not Friedman. For Friedman, the *ob* gene was a siren's call. It could lead the way to an understanding of the brain's system to control body weight. And that, of course, could lead to drugs that were directed at the brain system. They could be the first treatments that really did allow people to permanently lose weight. The seminal discovery was already made—*ob* mice were missing that crucial gene that is used to control eating and weight. He resolved to find the *ob* gene.

These days, molecular genetics has become so sophisticated that it would not take long to find the *ob* gene if you knew it was missing in *ob* mice, or so mutated that it was useless. There are detailed maps of mouse chromosomes and mouse genes publicly available on the Internet, and technology has allowed research that seemed completely infeasible just a few years ago. But Friedman began developing a strategy for finding the *ob* gene in the early 1980s, when the tools for molecular genetics were rudimentary and when no one had ever found a gene without first knowing what protein it coded for. Friedman knew what he needed to do. He had to find a way to progressively narrow down the area where the gene might lie on chromosome 6 until he was so close that he could seize the gene. And he had to be as clever and as efficient as possible.

The plan was developed with a team of scientists, including Rudy Leibel. It relied on a basic principle of genetics: When two genes are close together on a chromosome, they will be carried along in tandem for generation after generation. The closer they are to each other, the more tightly they will be linked. That is why, for example, people with red hair tend to have freckles—the red hair gene is close to the gene for freckles—and why there is no particular link between having red hair and being tall. Genes for height are nowhere near genes for hair color.

To find a gene like *ob*, you could look for known genes nearby that were inherited along with *ob*. The idea would be to find genes on either side of *ob* on chromosome 6 so that you bracket the *ob* gene. Then you would look for other genes inside the bracket, gradually closing in on *ob* until you were so close that you could start picking apart the region where *ob* must lie, looking for the particular gene that directs the brain to make the satiety factor.

In theory, it sounds straightforward. But what Friedman, Leibel, and the others in the group were attempting was the genetic equivalent of finding a needle in a haystack. They had no idea what the needle—the *ob* gene—would look like or what it did. All they knew was that it was not working in *ob* mice and that it was on chromosome 6.

The key to making the project work was to find the marker genes, which would serve as road signs, on either side of *ob*. The scientists needed a lot of them, and they needed genes that were easy to find. And they also needed a lot of animals, because the way to see whether genes are close together is to mate animals, generation after generation of animals, and ask whether the marker gene, the road sign, is inherited along with the gene of interest, in this case, the *ob* gene.

It was a daunting task—Friedman estimated that they needed to identify a 300-kilobase region, or 300,000 DNA bases, the chemical building blocks of DNA, out of the nearly 3 billion kilobases (3,000,000,000 bases) in the mouse genome. That would require eighteen hundred mice, half *ob* and half normal, just to start the breeding studies, and the studies would take years.

"At the time, this was arguably the most high-tech problem in science," Friedman says.

But he was not afraid. On December 9, 1986, he purchased his first animals. It was a step so momentous that he saved the purchase order, and he still has it.

"It begins with just an incredible sense of joy in those ways of thinking about what was wrong with this mouse. The technical opportunity and the fomenting excitement in this area were just unbelievable," he recalls. "I was naïve, of course. I started thinking about the excitement and the opportunity, and I didn't think early on about the management issues that would surface. There were so many logistical issues trying to build a project like this. It was hard. It was very, very hard. The problem was that I was overly optimistic about how long it would take. I had no idea how it would feel to be four, five years into the project. Everything was on the line, and I had no idea how it would end.

"The project unfolded as an empirical search for these probes," Friedman continued. He used every method known at the time. At one point he traveled with a graduate student to London so the student could learn a new technique for finding marker genes that involved slicing mouse chromosomes. His group then spent years searching for tiny stretches of DNA that can be identified because they are snipped by bacterial enzymes. That property could make them useful as markers.

And as the years crept by, Friedman became increasingly worried that it all would be for naught—some other lab would beat him to the prize, the identification of the *ob* gene. "I was so captivated and convinced that this was going to be important that I was sure there had to be other labs working on it," he said. "Over the years, I heard

about other groups trying—a Japanese group, a guy in the pharma-
ceutical industry, Jeff Flier [a Harvard researcher]."

But his greatest worry was that some other lab, looking around
in the mouse genome for some completely different gene, would just
stumble upon the *ob* gene by chance. Researchers might find a gene
for another trait on chromosome 6 and then, while they were focus-
ing on a narrow region of that chromosome 6, might ask, What other
genes are there? And, serendipitously, they might find the *ob* gene.

Friedman was haunted by this scenario. "You make an enormous
investment in this project. Then someone lands on your gene, and
you're blown up. This is a torturous way to live." He worried every
time his phone rang. "The first thing I thought of every time I got a
call from someone I didn't know: They've found *ob*."

And then, he said, he had another problem: Once you find two
markers bracketing *ob* so closely that you will not do better, how do
you actually find the gene in that chromosomal region? "You have
to make an inventory of all the genes in the region and ask which
one is different" in *ob* mice. There would be hundreds of thousands
of base pairs, maybe a million, to analyze, Friedman says, a task that,
at the time, seemed like it might not even be possible. "It's clear now
that it is possible. It's just pretty damn hard," he says.

By 1993, Friedman had his markers—he had found a region on
chromosome 6, 650,000 base pairs long, that contained the *ob* gene.
Now he just had to find it.

To do that, he proceeded systematically. He would find each gene
in the region by isolating distinctive small pieces of DNA that mark
the ends of genes. Then, having found a gene, he would examine it,
going gene by gene, to see if the gene was present and functioning in
normal mice but not in obese animals with the *ob* mutation.

Eventually, he came up with four possible genes in the region
where *ob* must reside. In each case, Friedman says, "we asked, 'Does
it make sense for it to be *ob*? Where is it usually expressed?'" One
gene turned out to direct cells to make an enzyme, inosine mono-
phosphate dehydrogenase, that was clearly not *ob*. This enzyme is
what scientists call a housekeeping enzyme: every cell in the body
needs it, and every cell makes it just to go about normal cellular
functions. When Friedman looked at cells from fat, and from the

brain, small intestine, stomach, pancreas, lung, heart, liver, spleen, and testes, all were using that gene.

Then he looked at another gene, which the group had labeled 2G7. It was used by fat cells. And not by any others. Friedman could hardly bear to hope. A picture was beginning to fit together, and it made perfect sense. Suppose 2G7 was it, the *ob* gene, the gene that was directing cells to make a satiety factor. Then you might expect the cells that were using 2G7 and making the protein it encoded to be fat cells. Fat cells, after all, are the repositories of fat. If you had enough to eat, if you wanted to send a signal to your brain to stifle your appetite, what better way than to have your fat cells do the signaling? The same thing could happen if you did not have enough to eat. You would have to use your stored fat for energy, and your fat cells would send a signal to your brain saying that more food was needed. Your brain would respond by making you eat.

But a nice theory was not enough. If 2G7 was the *ob* gene, it would have to pass a final test. Researchers would have to show that it was not working properly in the *ob* mouse.

Friedman devised the critical experiment.

That year, a new strain of obese mice had been found, known as *ob-2J*. The experiment would look at 2G7 in those mice, in the original *ob* mice, and in normal mice. To do that, the scientists would look at RNA, which is copied from active genes. They would use a test, known as the "Northern blot," that could quantify the amount of RNA made from 2G7. There were several possible outcomes: One was that the normal mice were making RNA from 2G7 and the two obese strains were not. That would mean 2G7 was the *ob* gene and that it was missing or completely inactive in the obese mice. That was why the obese mice were so fat.

Another possibility was that the normal mice were making RNA and one or both of the obese strains were making it too, but theirs was nonfunctional. That also would mean that 2G7 was *ob*. This time, though, the result would say that the *ob* mutation created a satiety signal that was a dud, completely ineffective.

The third possibility was that all three mice made normal amounts of perfectly functional RNA. Then 2G7 would not be the *ob* gene.

Friedman could hardly wait. As soon as possible, on Friday afternoon, May 6, 1994, a member of the research group, Margherita Maffei, set up the Northern blot test. Then she left for the day, planning to finish the experiment when she returned on Monday.

Friedman was tortured by the uncertainty. He could not bear to wait all weekend. So he called Maffei—he called her repeatedly—but she was gone, at a friend's wedding, and not answering her phone. "I left a message on her machine saying, 'Please come in,'" Friedman says. Maffei, who did not check her messages that weekend, had no idea.

"I needed to know the answer," Friedman said. Saturday evening, he returned to Rockefeller University, striding down the empty corridors to his lab. He poked through Maffei's refrigerator where she kept her reagents, found the experiment that she had started, took it out of her refrigerator, and set it up.

This experiment involved running an electrical current through a slab of gel, which would separate RNA molecules according to their charge. The RNA molecules were then transferred to a special paper that was labeled with a radioactive tracer, making them visible on X-ray film. You develop the images with the usual photographic developing solutions and then look for black spots, indicating radioactivity from RNA. If there was RNA at a particular position on the gel, there would be a black spot on the paper. If there was no protein, the paper would be blank in that position. The more RNA that was being made, the more radioactivity and the darker the spot on the paper.

Maffei had already run the RNA samples on the gel and transferred them to the special paper. What remained was for Friedman to expose the paper to a radioactive marker for the gene 2G7, wash the paper to remove the excess radioactivity so that any that remained would signal the gene attached to RNA, and expose the paper to the X-ray film. This typically takes most of a day, and Friedman finished at midnight.

With the experiment running, there was nothing more for Friedman to do. It would take all night to finish, and standing over it would not help. Restless, anxious, he went home.

"I couldn't sleep," Friedman says. He tossed in bed, his mind raced. Finally, he gave up all pretense of sleeping and at five in the

morning, he got out of bed, dressed, and dashed to the lab. He seized the photographic film, rushed it to the darkroom, dipped it into developer, set a timer, and waited, with a pounding heart. Hardly bearing to breathe, he lifted the film out of the bath of developer and looked. There it was. A small black spot corresponding to the RNA made by the normal mouse's fat cells. A very large dark spot, corresponding to massive overproduction of what must be defective RNA from the *ob* mouse's fat cells. And nothing at all, just a blank space, corresponding to a complete lack of RNA from the *ob-2J* mouse's fat cells.

"The second I saw this blot, I was certain," he said. He knew he had the *ob* gene. And, Friedman added, "I was pretty confident that it was a hormone that regulates weight." Everything had fallen into place. A decade of work, thousands of mice, the great gamble of his career, had paid off. He had found the gene.

And he was in awe. "Here is this simple hormone that solves the problem of how to track millions of calories over a lifetime."

He named the molecule "leptin," from the Greek word *leptos*, meaning "thin." "The idea is that in the absence of leptin, you're fat, so leptin keeps you thin," Friedman explains.

Friedman hung the film from that crucial Northern blot on the wall of his office, where it remains to this day.

Seeing that film in the gray light of early morning, alone in his silent lab, staring at the strip of shiny film, he says, "was the closest thing to a religious experience I ever had."

SIX MONTHS

Jerry Gordon never mentions free will at the diet group meeting just after Thanksgiving in 2004. It is only six months into the two-year study, but his initial euphoria is long gone. Those hopes he had over the summer of losing a pound or two a week, week in and week out, are beginning to look like pipe dreams. Not only is he no longer losing, but the weight is coming back, and he is starting to despair, and he blames only himself.

He speaks about his struggles with the low-calorie diet and how frustrating it is to still be fat eight months after the study began. But the discussion that night is, in a sense, all about free will. Does he have it or not? Is his eating a matter of choice, or is it driven by a brain that is not at all under his mind's command?

Jerry begins by saying he did not exercise much in the past week because he had a cold. And, he says, he ate—not something delicious and tempting, but raisin bran.

"I have a box of raisin bran that I snorted for a day and a half. Then I didn't buy it for, like, a week." Deciding he had gotten control of himself, Jerry bought the cereal again, but found himself dipping in, just like before. "I thought I was ready, but I wasn't." In itself, raisin bran is not so fattening, Jerry explains, but he just could not stay away. "The raisin bran is only about 125 calories for three-quarters of a cup, but like, you know, I'm doing two servings and then lying about an additional half a serving, and at nighttime I'm doing an additional serving."

What else went wrong? Well, he says, his wife bought his daughter some chocolate-covered almonds. That was during the week when there was no raisin bran in his house, and he felt he needed something sweet. "I managed to find my sweetness elsewhere. That was the chocolate-covered almonds."

At Thanksgiving, he had "stuffing, sweet potatoes, and wine, wine, wine." This happened, he explains, "because I was around my mother-in-law."

Leslie Womble looks down at Jerry's food record: "And what are the crackers you're eating?" Oh, those, he replies. "They're giant crackers. They're from Fresh Fields. They're, like, three-seeded. If you're a mouse or a bird, you would love them. They're not little crackers—they're about 6 inches by 2½ inches."

Jerry had tried several times to analyze why he was having so much trouble. He'd worked so hard to lose 45 pounds, and now he has gained 8 back.

"I'll be honest with you. I've often found myself eating to fuel myself. The nervous eating, the eating to get off the diet. If I'm not actively conscious of being on a diet and trying to accomplish a goal, it becomes very tough for me. It's like you're on the bus or you're not. After the sixth month or so, I kind of got tired of doing it. I still believed in it, but I started eating more. At the same time I still believe I will return to this on January 1, or so I am telling myself."

He wants desperately to be thin. He saw a photograph of himself taken at Thanksgiving, and he was appalled. "I still look fat as a bus. I'm already back to not being happy with my appearance. I'm disappointed, and I feel like I ran out of steam." He still tries to record his food, he still tries to stay with the program, but extra calories keep creeping in.

"I've had the same breakfast for the last seven months. The only thing that has changed is, I lie about the portions."

And why, another man in the group asks, does he lie about the portions? Jerry does not really answer. Instead, he tells how he lies, using a measuring cup to keep track of how much he is eating, but then sneaking some more. "It's, like, you pour cereal into the cup, and you take a fistful while you're at it."

Carmen Pirollo says he struggled, too, at times throwing caution to the wind, shutting off that little voice in his head that says maybe he really shouldn't be eating what he's eating, or maybe he really shouldn't be eating when he's eating, deciding not to record his every morsel of food even though he knows he is supposed to. And so he had to ask himself what was really going on.

"You have to be really motivated—and we were," he says of himself and his fellow dieters. "For six months we did very well. But can you maintain this sort of thing? I think it's very unrealistic. We just weren't able to do it."

And so, he says, despite the fact that he tells himself he is the master of his eating, "I don't have that kind of control." It's not just an excuse for self-indulgence, he's decided, and it's not just a rationalization for staying fat. It must be a deep mind-brain divide. It must be that free will, when it comes to eating, is an illusion.

"We believe we have it, we believe we control it, but then life gets in the way."

7

The Girl Who Had No Leptin

Like any other professionals, obesity researchers have their lore. And one of their favorite stories is about the girl who had no leptin.

She was born in 1989 to Pakistani parents who were living in England, and she seemed normal at birth. But by the time she was four months old, it was clear that something was seriously wrong with her appetite—she was insatiable. Whatever food she got, she ate, and whatever she ate was not enough. Her weight soared so that when she was a year old, she weighed 40 pounds, far above the fiftieth percentile for her age, which was 18 pounds, and 50 percent higher even than the ninety-eighth percentile for her age, which was 27 pounds, meaning that 98 percent of one-year-olds weighed no more than 27 pounds.

She continued to demand food, food, and more food, screaming and having tantrums when she was denied it. And her weight continued to climb. As she got heavier and heavier, her legs started to bow out from supporting her weight. Her doctors fixed that with knee surgery, but new problems arose as she continued to gain. When she was six years old, she weighed 130 pounds, twice the average for a child her age, and her thighs had gotten so big she could not plant her feet flat on the ground. She had liposuction on her thighs to enable her to walk again, yet all the while, she continued to eat and continued to grow fatter and fatter. At age eight, she weighed 190 pounds. The child's parents put a lock on the pantry.

But she foraged in trash cans and ate frozen fish sticks straight from the freezer.

The girl's doctors could not figure out what was wrong. The child did not have a brain tumor; her thyroid hormone levels were normal. There was one hint, however. Her uncontrollable urges to eat bore an uncanny resemblance to the behavior of *ob* mice. But until the little girl was five years old, no one knew what was making the *ob* mice so fat, to say nothing of knowing how to cure their massive obesity.

That changed on that Sunday morning in May 1994 when Jeff Friedman saw those telltale black spots on the X-ray film, the day he discovered leptin. This was the insight that would cure the little girl who could not stop eating.

Those were heady times, those months after the leptin discovery. It seemed possible that the obesity problem had been solved and that obesity might be akin to type 1 diabetes, a hormone deficiency disease. And, like this form of diabetes, which is controlled with insulin, obesity might be controlled with injections of leptin.

But first there was basic laboratory work to be done, and Friedman could hardly wait to get at it. He knew nothing yet about the ravenously hungry girl living in London, but he did know that the mice were telling him something important and, in those early days in the spring and summer of 1994, he was reeling from the giddy aftermath of his stupendous discovery.

With leptin, it seemed, the intricate brain circuits that control appetite might finally be unraveled. And that offered new hope for a solution to the problem that is the bane of every dieter. Most people find that there is a certain weight, which some obesity researchers call the "set point," that their body keeps returning to. They can diet; they can lose weight; they can feel that this time they really are in control. Yet vexingly, their weight inevitably drifts back up to where it started. Research studies of weight loss programs find the same thing: people can lose a lot of weight at first, but a year or two later, nearly everyone has gained everything back. At best, dieters can sustain, on average, a 5 to 10 percent weight loss.

force." Leptin would act like a spring, pulling you back to your old weight.

Still, at the time, as obesity researchers saw it, all the evidence pointed to an undeniably simple solution to the weight loss problem—leptin injections should make fat people thin. The hormone injections should act like a sort of "virtual fat," as Friedman put it. They would trick the brain into thinking the person had put on enough fat to provide that extra spurt of leptin. And just as blowing hot air onto a thermostat would make the thermostat turn off the furnace, giving a fat person leptin injections should make the brain shut down the appetite.

But tantalizing as the idea was, it was still a conjecture. Just because an idea made logical sense did not mean it would hold up in the bright light of rigorous scientific study. The first critical experiments lay ahead: What would happen if you gave leptin to a fat mouse, and what would happen if you gave the hormone to a normal mouse?

Friedman began by cleaning up the last loose ends from the original leptin experiment. What, he asked, had gone wrong with leptin in the *ob* mice? The large black spot on the gel showed they were making something with their leptin gene, but it was not working like leptin. Why not? The answer was that the leptin gene in *ob* mice had a fatal defect, a simple mutation about three-quarters of the way down that changed a single DNA building block from one chemical, cytosine, to another, thymidine. That created a stop signal in the synthesis of leptin so each leptin molecule was abruptly and prematurely terminated. The fat cells in the *ob* mice were making leptin fragments, and those fragments were duds, unable to function properly, unable to tell the animals' brains that it was time to stop eating. The result was the same as having no leptin at all.

Of course, the leptin discovery would be useless if the hormone only worked in mice. So before continuing his research, Friedman asked if humans made it, too. They did.

The real test of the leptin hypothesis, though, was to make enough leptin to use it as a drug in mice and then to inject it into mice to see if they lost weight. Making leptin was straightforward. The molecular biology revolution of the 1980s had taught scientists the trick.

But it is not just dieters whose weights stay within a narro
this happens to everyone, Friedman notes. In fact, weight c
so fine-tuned that it would be impossible without some ph
cal control mechanism. No one, he says, can consciously
food intake as precisely as the body does naturally. There i
reason why weight is so stable.

"The idea here is that there is something akin to a th
that regulates body fat," Friedman said. Instead of monitor
the fat thermostat in the brain would monitor leptin levels.
cells release the hormone into the blood, which carries
brain, the level of leptin in the blood reflects the amount
the body. Fat people might have the equivalent of a therm
is set too high, or that is malfunctioning so that it takes m
than normal for the brain to respond.

The hypothesis would equate the set point to the ten
setting on a thermostat. With the brain reading leptin level
a thermostat reads temperature levels, the brain, by makii
hungry or satiated, could control the body's fat levels to k
within a narrow range.

The idea of leptin as a signaler of body fat also provid
nations of why some people are naturally fatter than others.
is that some may have fat cells that are genetically dispose(
meager amounts of leptin. Their bodies would need more f
a strong enough leptin signal to the brain. Others may be g
predisposed to respond weakly to the hormone, perhap
the receptor molecules on their brain cells, where leptin
signals, only feebly bind leptin. They, too, would need m(
the brain to sense it had received the right amount of lept

The notion of leptin as a body fat regulator could als
why fat parents tend to have fat children and why the biolo
dren of thin parents often are thin. What may be inherited
ity of fat cells to make leptin at a particular rate or an abi
brain to respond to the hormone.

But, Friedman said, there could be many ways for lept
trol weight. "The way I think of it is, what leptin does is t
biological force," he explains. "The net result is to maint
within a range. The further you go in either direction, the g

Once you have a gene—and Friedman had the leptin gene—you splice it into bacteria and thereby turn the bacteria into little factories that squirt out the gene's protein. Jeff Halaas, a student in Friedman's lab, followed this recipe, got his leptin, and injected it into mice. They published the results in the journal *Science* in July 1995, showing that every prediction about leptin held true.

When Friedman and his colleagues gave leptin to *ob* mice, the animals lost 30 percent of their body weight in just two weeks, with no apparent side effects. The mice both ate less and increased their metabolism. Their body temperature rose, indicating they were burning calories at a faster rate, and they even moved around their cages like normal mice. Before they were treated with leptin, the *ob* mice looked like round balls of fur, their heads minuscule in comparison to their massive bodies. Afterward, almost overnight, they turned into sleek, lean creatures, with no outward sign that they had ever been so lumberingly fat.

Lean mice, too, lost weight when they received leptin injections, and the more leptin they received, the thinner they grew. When the researchers gave mice enough leptin to double the natural level of the hormone, the animals became like anorexics. They stopped eating and lost essentially all of their body fat in four days, going from 12.2 percent fat to 0.67 percent.

Other scientists were dumbfounded. "When you are talking about 0.67 percent body fat, that means that the animals have no adipose tissue," said Richard Atkinson, an obesity researcher who was then at the University of Wisconsin in Madison. Since about 1 percent of body fat is bound up in cell membranes, when the mice got down to 0.67 percent fat, "that means they completely got rid of their body fat."

In a paper published alongside Friedman's in *Science*, researchers led by L. Arthur Campfield of Hoffman-La Roche showed that leptin also worked when lean mice were made plump with a high-fat diet. With leptin injections, the mice immediately started eating half as much and quickly shed their excess weight.

Scientists were ecstatic.

Philip Gordon, who was then the director of the National Institute of Diabetes and Digestive and Kidney Diseases in Bethesda, Maryland, said that in terms of weight control, the leptin discovery was "one of the most important observations that's been made in recent times.

"We have to press this issue as rapidly as we can," he said.

The leptin discovery, said Theodore Van Itallie, the long-time obesity researcher at Columbia University's College of Physicians and Surgeons in New York, "could be an absolutely extraordinary advance in understanding why some people are vulnerable to obesity."

Mickey Stunkard called the results "fabulous."

Of course, drug companies could hardly wait to start developing leptin. Not only did it look as though it might be the first obesity drug in history that actually worked, but it had another advantage. For drug companies, the perfect weight loss drug would be one that a person would have to take for life or risk getting fat again. And that, it seemed, was leptin. The experiments with mice indicated that lost weight would be regained if the leptin treatments were discontinued. Should the same hold true in humans, overweight people might need to take leptin permanently in order to stay thin.

So Rockefeller University, which owned the rights to the leptin gene, asked companies to start bidding. The winner was Amgen, which paid the astonishingly high price of $20 million and agreed to pay many times that amount if the hormone proved useful in treating fat people. Friedman had hoped that Rockefeller would award the rights to a different company, Millennium Pharmaceuticals, which he had helped found. But he did well with the Amgen agreement—he and his team got nearly $7 million of the $20 million, and a bit less than half of that money went to him. The university, Friedman says, determined who got what. The money, he adds, was not the prime motivator. "I'd have done it for free," Friedman said.

Other companies saw room to develop their own drugs. They might find variations of leptin that were more effective, or drugs that prompted the body to make leptin, for example.

Amgen began its leptin study in April 1997. Two and a half years later, in October 1999, the results appeared in the *Journal of the American Medical Association*.

They were not what scientists expected.

It was a preliminary study, involving fifty-four people of normal weight and seventy-three who were obese, weighing, on average, 198 pounds. The participants were randomly assigned to inject themselves once a day with leptin or, as a control, saline solution. Then the study continued with just the obese subjects to assess leptin's ability to induce weight loss. All the obese patients, whether they were getting leptin or saline, were also asked to follow a weight loss diet that gave them 500 fewer calories a day than they needed to keep their weight constant. If they followed the diet, they should lose a pound a week, with or without leptin.

The diet, as might be expected, did not help much. In twenty-four weeks, the participants taking the placebo instead of leptin and trying to diet lost an average of 3 pounds.

But the surprise was that leptin had little effect except at the highest dose tested, when two out of eight patients lost about 35 pounds each in twenty-four weeks. The others lost much less, and one gained nearly 20 pounds. The eight taking the highest leptin dose were the remnants of a group of eighteen assigned to take it; the rest dropped out after a month, complaining that they could not stand to inject themselves with several tablespoons a day of a substance that irritated their skin—making it itchy, red, and inflamed—and was painful to administer.

Now, with the reversal of fortune for leptin, obesity researchers were unsparing in their comments.

"You would have to look at it and say there has not yet been any convincing evidence that this is a therapeutic benefit in anything other than a minor fraction of patients," said Jeffrey S. Flier, chief of endocrinology at the Beth Israel Deaconess Medical Center in Boston.

"The great hope for leptin has not held up," Jules Hirsch, at Rockefeller University, said. "It doesn't look to me like what's wrong with human beings is a deficit of leptin."

Jeff Friedman saw some hope—it looked like a subset of people might respond to leptin injections and lose weight. But Amgen quickly lost interest in leptin as a miracle treatment for millions of fat people.

The question, though, was, Why didn't the obese people in Amgen's study respond to leptin? The possibility, or perhaps the *likelihood*, was that leptin was not their problem. These people were making plenty of leptin—they were not the human equivalent of the *ob* mice. And since adding more leptin did not make them lose weight, it must be that the hormone was being blocked from acting somewhere along its passage from the fat cells to the appetite-controlling pathways in the brain. Leptin might not be getting into the brains of some people, or there could be a problem along the brain pathways that are signaled when cells respond to leptin. In either case, obstructions before or after leptin reached its target in the brain would mean that giving more leptin could have little or no effect on a person's weight. The challenge now was to unravel the entire leptin pathway, from its release by fat cells to the cascade of signals set off when it gets into the brain. Leptin might not be the magic weight loss drug, but it could be the lever to pry open a portal to developing drugs that really work.

"Most look at the discovery of leptin as the seminal event," Steve Heymsfield said. The pathways from the body to the brain and within the brain that so exquisitely control how much is eaten and how much a person weighs are, he said, "like a jigsaw puzzle." With leptin, he added, "suddenly there was a puzzle to put together."

So the leptin story moved back into the research labs, where scientists reasoned that the trick to curing obesity will be to understand so well the brain's control of eating that it will be possible to find safe and effective ways to disrupt it.

It did not take long for the puzzle to start filling in. Within a few years, increasingly complex and eye-glazing diagrams began appearing in scientific journals as researchers discovered more and more chemicals and neurons that are part of the body's system to control when and how much we eat. The diagrams typically used different colors for different nerve circuits and featured arrows going back and forth between nerve cells and peptides—small protein fragments—with impenetrable names.

The nerve pathways, like the Dr. Dolittle animal the pushmi-pullyu, work at cross-purposes—eat or don't eat. It is the balance between these pathways that determines whether you are hungry and when you are satisfied. And leptin affects both sides of the equation, stimulating pathways that make you feel satisfied and blocking those that make you want to eat. Its effects begin when fat cells release leptin and the hormone is swept into the brain. Washing over the entire brain, leptin attaches itself to cells mainly in one area, the arcuate nucleus of the hypothalamus, that central area on the underside of the brain that has long been known to be associated with control of eating. There, the hormone starts a nerve cell fusillade.

Part of the intricate system, scientists discovered, includes a barrage of peptides that signal nerve cells in the brain to amplify the leptin signal. Leptin strikes nerves in the hypothalamus that synthesize the hormone pro-opiomelanoctorin (POMC). The cells respond by breaking off some POMC to form a peptide, melanocyte-stimulating hormone, or MSH. That peptide in turn travels to other nerves, which results in a chain reaction that ends up as a feeling that you just can't take another bite of food.

At the same time, leptin blocks nerve pathways that make you want to start eating and ones that make you feel hungry. To do this, the hormone obstructs nerve cells in the hypothalamus that release appetite-stimulating chemicals with names like "agouti-related protein" and "neuropeptide Y." The result is that you no longer want to eat.

But the more scientists studied leptin, the more the hormone surprised them. At first they thought that it acted like most other hormones—attaching itself to brain cells and altering their function. Then they discovered that leptin can do something else. It can actually change the brain's wiring diagram, strengthening circuits that inhibit eating and weakening ones that spur the appetite. It can exert this effect at a critical period early in life, perhaps influencing appetite and obesity in adults. And, in adulthood, leptin can again alter the brain's wiring, permanently changing an animal's appetite and weight.

The work was in animals, but it amazed researchers. It might mean that there are critical times in infancy or childhood when a person's fate, to be fat or not, is sealed. That may be why some people start out thin and suddenly start to gain when they are three, four, or five years old, setting the stage for a lifetime of obesity. This may not be the complete story—the brain's weight-control mechanisms keep turning out to be much more subtle and much more complicated than anyone expects—but it certainly was provocative. It implied that if leptin acts in some people as it does in animals, rewiring the brain in adults, that might explain why some people, like Carmen Pirollo, start out skinny as a reed and then, like their parents and grandparents before them, grow fat in adulthood.

Weight loss centers hear such stories over and over again, of people who seemed born to be fat and others who say fatness just sneaked up on them.

At the University of Pittsburgh Medical Center's weight-management program, on a July day in 2004, a group of dieters shared their stories, all too familiar to those in the weight loss field.

There was Janet Forton, a rosy-cheeked professional woman who says she succeeded in every aspect of her life except weight control. She'd been fat since infancy and plagued by comparisons with her nonidentical twin sister. "The only day I weighed less than my sister is the day I was born. I breathed in, started putting on weight, and never stopped. My twin has never had a weight problem."

There was Mary Frances Neely, age forty-five, with fair skin, dark hair, brilliant blue eyes, and a body that was, clearly, fat. She said she'd been fat for her entire life, and her stories of struggling to lose almost defy the laws of biology.

"My journey started at birth. I was a fat baby, a fat child, a fat teenager." Her mother and her mother's relatives were obese; her father and many of his relatives had weight problems. "I wouldn't call them obese, just large."

When Neely was fourteen, she went on her first serious diet, going to Weight Watchers with her mother. But the 80 pounds she lost came right back. "From then on, it was just a barrage of gaining and losing. The cabbage diet, the grapefruit diet, just about any diet you could name, my mother and I did it. I would lose massive amounts of weight. And then it would come right back on." She felt like a failure—everyone else she knew was thin, and it was hard to believe that after all the effort she put into losing weight, she could not stay thin afterward. So she tried again; she tried harder. In college, she resorted to a semi-starvation diet. "I had cigarettes and black coffee, and I would eat things like a salad with no salad dressing." Her weight started to plummet, finally sinking to 140 pounds from over 200.

"It was the first time in my adult life that I had lost more than 100 pounds. I was in the worst physical shape that I had ever been in. I was tired, I didn't have any energy. My skin was real pasty-looking. My nails wouldn't grow and they split." But, she says, "I was ecstatic because I had lost the weight. Of course, I gained the weight back."

And that became the pattern of her life—diet, lose weight, lose control, gain it back. "I have lost 600 or 700 pounds in my adult lifetime," Neely says. The last time she tried an extreme diet was eight years before, and she lost more than 100 pounds. She was determined to keep it off, but doing so meant a life of constant deprivation. She describes a weight-maintenance diet that, she says, allowed her about 600 calories a day. She would have fruit in the morning, a salad with no dressing for lunch, and the same salad along with a grilled chicken breast for dinner. She also exercised, spending an hour and twenty minutes at the gym five days a week. But although this sounds like the life of an anorexic, Neely was not thin. Her weight was normal; no one would look at her and say she was underweight. Yet, she insists, if she let up, even if she skipped a few days at the gym, she would start to gain weight. She maintained her vigilance for five years. Then she loosened her iron control, and the weight came back.

She thought about having surgery to lose weight, but hesitated. "I wanted to try to do it myself, one more time." So she went to a doctor who put her on a low-carbohydrate diet. In nine months she lost 20 pounds. Her doctor was happy, but Neely despaired. She was hungry all the time. She was trying every trick in the diet book—when you're a fat person, you have been on so many diets that you know all the advice, you could write the diet books, she says. "Instead of a dinner plate I would use a salad plate. Instead of a bowl, I used a ramekin. Everything I downsized." But she still weighed more than 300 pounds, and her life was impossible. She hated being fat.

"I have a teenage daughter, and I could not go with her to an amusement park. I knew I could not fit into the ride seats, and I did not want to embarrass her." She wanted to exercise; she knew it would be good for her. But her hips ached from the extra weight, so much, she says, that when she got up in the morning, she couldn't walk. She worried about her health: "I had diabetes, I had high blood pressure, I had bladder incontinence, and I didn't think I was that old."

A 20-pound weight loss had made no difference to her health or her life. She looked no different. Also, she says, "my blood sugar did not come down. None of that changed." Suppose she kept up a steady weight loss of 20 pounds every nine months: it would take years to become thin. "I had over 150 pounds to lose."

It is not, of course, that Neely never ate and somehow got fat. Instead, it is that every time she lost weight, she would eventually slip up and start to eat. Once she started, she could not stop. It was behavior that seemed so bizarre she sought professional help.

"I've even gone to a psychiatrist," Neely says. "My problem is that I'm never full. I could eat two Big Macs, a supersized fries, supersized Cokes, two milkshakes, and I would not feel full."

To a research scientist, such stories do not indicate psychiatric problems. Instead, they point to powerful biological effects that almost certainly, in one way or another, involve the brain circuits revealed by the discovery of leptin.

Dr. Stephen O'Rahilly of Addenbrooke's Hospital in Cambridge, England, who studies genetic causes of extreme obesity, was struck by the story that Neely told. He's heard ones like it so many times. People start out telling how they lived on chicken breasts and 600 calories a day, how they put their dinner on a salad plate. And then, finally, they reveal their secret shame, the insatiable urge to eat, the feeling of never being full despite the Big Macs and the supersized fries and the Cokes and the milkshakes. Fat people are fat because their drive to eat is very different from the drive in thin people, O'Rahilly says. And that is something thin people never understand.

"A lot of thin people think that because they can skip a meal and feel a bit hungry, everyone can do the same. They assume the sensation of hunger is the same for everyone." O'Rahilly says he knows from his own research and from personal experience that it is not. He's not massively obese but he is heavy, and hunger for him is not just a mild sensation. "I never skip lunch," O'Rahilly says. "I just can't." Hunger makes him feel terrible—"like an Antichrist," he says.

The discovery of leptin's effects early in life, at least in animals, came because two scientists—Richard B. Simerly and Sebastian G. Bouret at the Oregon Primate Research Center in Beaverton—noticed that leptin seemed eerily similar to what they knew about sex hormones, such as estrogen and testosterone. During brain development, there is a surge in these sex hormones that alters the very circuitry of the brain, shaping it so that the brains of males turn out to be very different from the brains of females. That sort of change was what the two researchers studied, and they had thought it was restricted to the effects of sex hormones. Then they saw a paper on leptin, by Jeff Flier at Harvard Medical School, reporting that there is a surge of leptin early in life, at least in mice.

"Bingo," Simerly said. "The lights went on."

They decided to look first at adult *ob* mice, which make no functioning leptin and so would not have had that leptin surge. In those mice, the nerve connections in the arcuate nucleus of the hypothalamus were weak, the scientists found, an intriguing discovery because that part of the brain develops soon after birth.

That led Simerly to ask whether he could alter those connections by giving *ob* mice a surge of leptin early in life, mimicking what happens in normal mice. The plan worked—the leptin surge reshaped the connections in the hypothalamus, making their brains look like the brains of normal mice.

Then Friedman and his colleagues discovered that leptin surges when the brain is developing were only part of the way that leptin shapes the brain. It also can rewire the brain almost instantaneously.

Their discovery arose when they looked at the nerve connections in brain slices from *ob* mice. The animals had strong circuits in the pathways in the arcuate nucleus that stimulate eating. But the circuits that decrease appetite were weak. Then they gave the animals leptin. Within six hours, their brain circuits were like those in normal animals. Two days later, the mice lost their huge appetites.

The researchers then tested another hormone, ghrelin, a peptide whose effects are the opposite of leptin's, giving it to normal mice. Four days later, the animals were eating more and their brains were rewired in the opposite direction. Friedman was taken aback. Never had he imagined that the brain's circuitry was so fluid.

"I'd always imagined this system had a fixed architecture, like a plumbing system," he said. "A certain number of pipes were laid out or fixed." He said he had thought the flow of signals in the hypothalamus was regulated by the equivalent of opening or closing valves. But that was not what happened.

"In this case, the brain is adding and subtracting pieces of pipe. Nerves are not appearing or disappearing, but the way they are connected to each other is," Friedman said.

The obvious next question, of course, is whether human brains are shaped by leptin surges and, if so, whether the hormone might be determining if a person is destined to be fat or thin. "Leptin acts on the brain to regulate food intake," Simerly said. "If the brain pathway isn't there or is greatly reduced, you would expect that process to be deficient. Your brain is perhaps not sensing how fat you are."

Many obesity researchers think that what was happening in mice is likely to be happening in humans. Jeff Flier likened the effects of leptin to brain changes when memories are stored. The brain almost seemed to be developing a memory for the weight it wanted the animal to be, which raises intriguing possibilities about weight regulation in people.

"It all comes back to the same issues—the whole issue of appetite and weight regulation in humans," Flier says. "It is at the interface of free will and determinism. There is certainly a strong biological underpinning to our drive to eat and maintain certain weights. We knew that before and we still know it. But now there is another layer of mechanisms by which things like hormones not only can affect the neurochemistry that affects how hungry you are but also can affect the wiring of your brain."

With leptin as the wedge to start prying open the secrets of weight control, scientists began describing in detail the long-term signals to regulate weight and short-term signals that act after each meal or snack to tell you that you've had enough or that you should keep eating or that it is time to eat again.

For example, scientists began paying more attention to ghrelin, which is released by the stomach when the stomach is empty, travels through the blood to the brain, and prods nerves in the hypothalamus that make the appetite-stimulating peptides. Those peptides act on the brain's eating-control pathways, with the result that when your stomach is empty, you want to eat. Jeff Friedman had used ghrelin in his brain-wiring studies as a sort of anti-leptin. But leptin is not the only thing that counters ghrelin. Another is peptide YY, or PYY, a peptide that is sent out from the gastrointestinal tract to reflect the calorie content of a meal. PYY blocks the nerves that are stimulated by ghrelin. The more calories you consume, the more is released. And the more you release, the more full you feel. That is why you eventually feel sated.

As they discovered these signaling systems, researchers—and drug companies—began asking whether these systems could be used to develop weight-control drugs. The possibilities just kept multiplying. For example, Dr. Gregory S. Barsh, of Stanford University, focused on agouti-related protein, or AgRP, a peptide in the cascade that makes animals eat. Leptin blocks its actions, making animals stop eating. To see what might be possible, Barsh injected mice with a drug that mimics AgRP. The results astounded him—a single injection made the animals gorge for a week. And if he gave the mice another drug that blocked AgRP, they immediately stopped eating.

"We think it helps control the long-term energy balance," Dr. Barsh said. "In one 24-hour period, you or I may eat half of what we eat in another 24-hour period. But over the long term our body fat remains stable. So there needs to be a mechanism to account for that stability. Or supposing you went on a drastic diet for three or four days. There will be a drive to eat; you feel hungry. Where does that drive come from?" The regulator, Dr. Barsh suggests, could be agouti-related protein.

But PYY, the anti-leptin, also counteracts AgRP. (Actually, the PYY that is an appetite suppressor is not the complete PYY peptide. PYY starts out as a chain of thirty-six amino acids. Cells chop off the first three, and what's left is PYY_{3-36}. That is the part that suppresses appetite. The complete PYY, with those first three amino acids on the chain, can actually *increase* food intake. This seems impossibly complex, but it is what happens.) The thought, though, was that if AgRP makes animals eat, then PYY_{3-36}, which blocks it, should make animals, or people, stop eating. Or so reasoned Dr. Stephen R. Bloom, a professor of endocrinology at Hammersmith Hospital at Imperial College School of Medicine in London.

PYY$_{3-36}$ seemed perfect—it is released by the intestines after a meal, overweight people make less of it than thin people, and studies in animals indicated it might be the body's signal for satiety. People who have bariatric surgery, which reduces the size of the stomach, make more, and of course they often say their appetite is greatly diminished.

The rat studies were a bit tricky, Bloom reports, because the substance does not work if the animals are stressed. Stress, like PYY, turns off appetite, and it does so by acting on exactly the same nerve circuit that is hit by PYY. "If you make a big noise or pick up a rat or a mouse, it doesn't eat," Bloom says. And with those nerve circuits inhibited, PYY cannot inhibit them any more. That might explain why people often lose their appetite when they are under stress. Their brain circuits that tell them they are hungry are blocked. But this can make it hard to do animal studies because you have to be sure that the rats are not stressed, and simply handling a rat stresses it. So Bloom had to carefully prepare the rats, getting them used to being picked up and given a sham injection—with saline in this case—often enough that they became indifferent to the procedure and ate normally afterward. Then he could ask whether PYY injections made the animals stop eating. They did. Now Bloom asked, would PYY make people stop eating?

Bloom's motivation for these studies was that he was saddened by the obese people he sees every day in his clinic. "Medically, it's a disaster to be obese," he said, and he saw suffering that went far beyond the medical problems he could treat. "The rate of suicide is doubled; they are unhappy; they have a lower average wage; they don't get married. They are unhappy people dying of nasty complications, and it's particularly sad because society tries to blame them."

He had spent years trying to see whether he could find reliable ways to trick people into eating less. But hoary methods like filling up with water or with bulky, low-calorie foods such as cabbage turned out to be useless—his subjects ate just as much over the course of a day. He tried infusing nutrients directly into the bloodstream, but his subjects were as hungry as ever.

That ruled out the two obvious causes of satiation, Bloom concluded: "It is neither from the food in circulation after it is absorbed nor from the fullness of the gut." Despite the exhortations of diet gurus who tell people to down cup after cup of water or have a bowl of soup or nibble on celery between meals so that they keep something in their stomachs, Bloom's careful studies showed such measures make no difference. Your appetite is the same. And that really should be no surprise, Bloom says. The brain's regulatory systems are too sophisticated for such simple ruses.

"Most of us are the same weight year after year," Bloom said. "We might be overweight, but we are the same weight year in and year out. Yet every day you are faced with this or that amount of food. You don't measure it; you just naturally regulate your food intake." Yet there was hope for PYY, he thought. It might be a signal in humans that the body has had enough food, in the short term at least, and so it, unlike something like celery or soup, might actually diminish people's appetites.

To find out, Bloom did a small study to see what would happen when he gave PYY to people. His subjects were twenty-four volunteers: half the subjects were men, and half were women; half were fat, and half were thin. They all came to the hospital at 8:30 a.m., and half of the volunteers got an injection of PYY while the rest, as a control, got an injection of saline. Neither the subjects nor the scientists who observed them knew who got the drug and who got the placebo. At 11:00 a.m., the investigators ushered the subjects over to a buffet lunch and watched how much they ate.

"It was dramatic," Bloom says. On average, those who had received PYY ate 30 percent less. And PYY, he adds, worked on everyone. "We haven't had anyone who didn't get a result." In fact, the effect lasted all day, with the obese people eating only 1,810 calories as compared with 2,456 for those given a saline injection. Even the thin people ate less—1,533 calories after they had the hormone infusion, but 2,312 when they had saline.

The PYY study was preliminary, but so promising that it was published by the prestigious *New England Journal of Medicine* on September 4, 2003. But going from a pilot study to a drug that works is a long process. Bloom says that as much as he would like to develop obesity drugs, he has limited funds as an academic. He started a small company, Thiakis; applied for a so-called use patent to develop PYY, which was already in the public domain and so not patentable as a hormone; and sold those rights to another company, Nastech, which then sold them to Merck. Merck, in turn, promised to pay more than $50 million if PYY ended up as a drug that is marketed. But in March 2006, Merck returned the rights to Nastech, saying that PYY had not been effective in its preliminary studies. Nastech said it will continue to develop the drug for the treatment of obesity.

But questions remain. For example, what if PYY, taken repeatedly, simply makes you feel ill, nauseated, rather than full? It can be hard to tell in preliminary studies whether a substance is reducing appetite by making an animal want to eat less or by making it feel so sick that it cannot eat. Most drugs fail in their preliminary studies in humans, and of course PYY would only be worth developing if it suppressed appetite but had no other effects.

In the meantime, Bloom switched his attention to another promising peptide known as oxyntomodulin. It's made in the small intestine, and its level increases after a meal. And the more you eat, the higher the blood levels of oxyntomodulin. The blood transports the peptide to the brain, where it inhibits the same brain circuits that are inhibited by PYY. In theory, oxyntomodulin should stifle the appetite.

Bloom tried it out with rats. In contrast to PYY, which resulted in about a 30 percent decrease in the amount of food the animals ate, oxyntomodulin shut down their eating entirely. But the hormone is much shorter-acting—rats that got oxyntomodulin stopped eating for a few hours, while PYY shut down their eating for a day.

People who have diseases like celiac disease or chronic pancreatitis, in which it would be detrimental to eat very much, turn out to have elevated levels of PYY and oxyntomodulin in their blood, Bloom noticed. And, he said, these people tend to be very thin and to complain that they have no appetite.

The same is true for obese people who have had gastric bypass surgery in order to lose weight. At first, Bloom said, when the surgery seemed so effective, researchers thought it was because patients could no longer absorb food. But it turned out that the malabsorption lasted just three or four days, after which the patients began absorbing nutrients farther down in the bowel than normal. "Their digestion was completely normal," Bloom says. So if malabsorption was supposed to elicit weight loss, "the procedure appears to be a complete failure."

Yet the patients continued to lose weight. They say they lose their appetite after the surgery, and it turns out, Bloom says, that these patients are releasing large amounts of PYY and oxyntomodulin. That means that if these two hormones really are the clue to the success of bariatric surgery, it may be possible someday to simulate the effects of the operation without doing the surgery.

In the meantime, Bloom did the same sort of study with oxyntomodulin as he did with PYY. Subjects agreed to inject themselves with the peptide or with saline, as a control, and their food intake was monitored. Over four weeks, those taking oxyntomodulin lost an average of $4\frac{1}{2}$ pounds without realizing that they were eating less.

"We felt pretty pleased," Bloom says. "We proved the principle."

And he knows how high the stakes are for people who are obese. He recently saw an acquaintance and was struck by how much weight the man had lost. What happened? Bloom asked. "He said, 'I've had a gastric bypass. It's wonderful. I just don't feel hungry anymore.'" The man, Bloom says, had been a social outcast, but now, with his weight loss, he had gotten married, and his wife had just had a baby. "No one had thought him attractive before," Bloom says.

While Bloom was doing his studies, Stephen O'Rahilly in Cambridge was conducting a parallel line of research with children. His work had actually begun even earlier, a few years before leptin was discovered, at a time when O'Rahilly was not thinking about specializing in obesity. His focus was on diabetes and, in particular, on unusual forms of the disease. Then a woman was referred to him because she had symptoms of an endocrine disorder: She was shaky and sweaty after meals. She had low levels of blood sugar, insulin, and cortisol. She was always tired. She never went through puberty. And she was incredibly fat.

O'Rahilly and his colleagues discovered the woman's problem— she had a genetic mutation in something called the prohormone convertase gene, which is necessary for processing a variety of hormones. That was why she had symptoms of an endocrine disorder.

It was also why she was so fat. Without that enzyme, her cells could not chop POMC into MSH. And without MSH, she never felt satiated, no matter how much she ate. A similar defect in mice also leads to obesity.

Hearing of O'Rahilly's work with the fat woman, a clinical geneticist in Oxford called him to ask if he would take a look at two fat children. They were huge, enormously obese, and the geneticist could not figure out what was wrong. By then, Jeff Friedman's paper had just been published, and O'Rahilly had just read it. When he heard about the children's symptoms, he said, "I got very excited." They sounded just like the *ob* mice's. These children, he decided, might be fat because they made no leptin.

It turned out that he was right, and one of those patients was the girl who had no leptin, the child who weighed 190 pounds when she was just eight years old and whose parents had had to put a lock on the pantry. She could actually be cured once leptin was discovered. She began receiving leptin shots when she was nine years old, a daily injection each morning at 8:00 a.m.

She became the first success, the first proof that it is possible to correct a genetic defect and thereby cure obesity.

To study the hormone's effects, O'Rahilly, his colleague Dr. I. Sadaf Farooqi, and others in O'Rahilly's group did a formal experiment. They put a digital scale in the girl's home so her family could weigh her every day and record her weight. They investigated her appetite by giving her a test meal, a lunch buffet of 1,650 calories after she had been fasting since breakfast. They measured her metabolic rate and her physical activity.

Before she began treatment, the little girl had a normal metabolic rate and normal activity level. But her behavior toward food was anything but normal. She quickly devoured the test meal. And she still was not satisfied, complaining afterward that she was hungry and asking for more to eat. After a week of leptin injections, she was a changed person, eating no more than her siblings, eating at the same speed as her siblings instead of gobbling her food, no longer demanding food between meals. Her weight plummeted.

"It was incredibly dramatic," O'Rahilly said. "This was a child who had never lost weight in her life." Her weight chart, he said, looked like Mount Everest, a steady sharp climb upward and, when her leptin treatments began, an equally sharp plummet.

Before taking leptin, the child was so distorted by fat that she appeared to have no neck; her arms were pushed out by her huge trunk, her belly hung over her groin, and her legs were so encased in fat that there was little sign of her knees. Afterward, she was a slender, graceful girl with a pointed chin, pronounced cheekbones, and shapely legs. She bore no resemblance to the grotesquely obese child she once had been.

The girl continues to take leptin, and she has effortlessly maintained her normal weight. Since then, O'Rahilly and Farooqi have treated four other children with what he calls "fantastic results"— leptin is curing them, just as it cured the first child.

Even adults responded. In one study, Dr. Julio Licinio of the University of California at Los Angeles and Dr. Metin Ozata from Gulhane Haydarpasa Training Hospital in Acibadem-Istanbul and their colleagues gave leptin to three adults, siblings from Turkey, who lacked it—a twenty-seven-year-old man and two women, one thirty-five years old and one forty. Within a week of treatment, their weights began to plummet. By the end of the eighteen-month study, these people, who had been enormously fat, became almost slender, normal-looking. The man lost 168 pounds, or 54 percent of his body weight. One woman lost 105 pounds, which was 43.5 percent of her body weight, and the other woman lost 132 pounds, which was 44.5 percent of her body weight. They went, O'Rahilly says, "from astonishing weights to complete normality."

O'Rahilly and Farooqi, though, who have treated only children so far, have had a disappointment. They encountered a child with no leptin in Pakistan. She was so hugely fat at age twelve that she could not walk and was confined to her bed. She died before O'Rahilly and Farooqi could treat her, succumbing to a respiratory infection. O'Rahilly explained that severe obesity, leading to a life spent mostly in bed, impairs breathing. That, combined with an immune defect that arises from a lack of leptin, "contributed to the tragic early death of this child."

While they were treating people who lacked leptin, O'Rahilly and Farooqi began searching for other obese children who might have genetic disorders. They put out a call to doctors worldwide to refer such children to them, reasoning that body weight is largely inherited. If it is inherited, then it involves genes. If it involves genes, then it will be easiest to start searching for those genes by finding people with the most severe genetic defects, those with the most pronounced obesity. And that means that one good place to start looking is in children with serious and intractable weight problems.

That, says O'Rahilly, is a classic tactic in medicine: Find people with extreme medical conditions. Identify pronounced genetic defects that caused those conditions. Then look for less severe defects among those in the general population who have less severe forms of the medical problem.

He has no doubt that body weight is, to a large extent, inherited. He cites the family studies, twins studies, and studies of adopted twins by Mickey Stunkard and others, saying they establish the role of inheritance beyond any doubt. "You really can't ignore that data," he says. "It's very powerful. And we've known about it for years and years."

Of course, he hastens to add, the genes that make people fat need an environment in which food is cheap and plentiful, the same way that genes that make people tall need an environment in which children are well nourished. Jeff Friedman likes to point out that people today are at least 3 inches taller on average than they were in the Civil War era—genes did not change in the interim, but the environment did. Now children in this country almost always get enough food for their genes to direct them to grow to their maximum height. The situation is likely to be the same with weight. These days, children, and adults, can easily get enough food for their genes to direct them to grow as fat as they can be.

But despite the studies dating back twenty years and more showing that genes determine body weight, O'Rahilly says, "the genetic study of obesity is in its infancy. It's twenty years behind cancer, ten years behind diabetes." The reason, he says, is that until recently there was no good way to get at those genes. Scientists needed a road map and a starting place. Now, he says, they have those, and the study of the genetics of obesity has begun attracting scientists like him. "With the discovery of leptin, it became more interesting."

So O'Rahilly and Farooqi studied children who got very fat when they were very young. Before long, they discovered four previously unknown genetic disorders, all affecting the brain pathways that were mapped with the discovery of leptin.

The most common so far is melanocortin-4 receptor deficiency. Those children may as well be making no leptin at all, because the leptin they make cannot signal them to stop eating. The details of the condition were clear from the animal work that mapped brain circuits that control eating. In these children, fat cells secrete leptin to tell the brain how fat the child is. The leptin enters the brain and stimulates POMC neurons in the hypothalamus. Those neurons in turn send out a chemical signal, alpha melanocyte-stimulating hormone, or MSH, to the next group of neurons in the cascade of reactions. But here the process breaks down for these children. They have a gene mutation that destroys the brain receptors for MSH, so even though leptin appropriately stimulates their POMC neurons, the signaling breaks down from there.

The children are tall and very fat. Although their metabolic rates were normal, they ate three times as much as their normal-weight brothers and sisters. Some had a partial loss of the gene's function. They were fat, but not as fat as children who had a total loss of the gene.

Not only did O'Rahilly and Farooqi find children with this genetic defect, but they discovered the defect is fairly common. They've studied over two thousand children with severe obesity and learned that 5 percent, or about one hundred of them, are obese because they have a melanocortin-4 receptor deficiency. And, starting with those children, they've traced the gene through family members and found hundreds of other people with the gene defect. "In England alone, there are likely to be thousands and thousands of patients with this disorder," O'Rahilly says.

By now, O'Rahilly and Farooqi have found children with genetic defects at every step of the leptin pathway.

They also addressed the question of why the children are so fat. Some obesity researchers have said that thin people are more fidgety and can eat without gaining weight because they burn more calories with their constant motion. They have suggested that fat people make an effort to mimic the naturally thin, trying to move about more, even trying to fidget, to burn a few extra calories. So are the obese children with genetic defects fat because they are slothful and are not burning many calories, or are they fat because they eat more than other people? O'Rahilly asked.

To find out, O'Rahilly and Farooqi kept the children away from food overnight and then provided them with what they call an "infinite breakfast," a buffet with so much food laid out that no one could eat it all. They observed how much the fat children ate and how much their normal-weight brothers and sisters ate.

"There may be subtle energy differences," O'Rahilly says, "but what's not so subtle is that these obese children eat much more than normal siblings. A two-year-old ate 2,000 calories—that's a day's calories for an adult."

It made sense, he noted: "These genes are expressed in or act on the hypothalamus, the area of the basal forebrain that acts on energy balance. In all cases, the dominant effect is on food intake. Not metabolism but behavior. These children are simply not satisfied."

O'Rahilly knows his conclusions make some people uncomfortable. "People don't like the genetics of behavior." And, he says, some gene enthusiasts have exaggerated the effects of genetics, claiming that virtually every human behavior is the result of a gene. "There is not likely to be a simple genetic explanation for not paying taxes or cheating on your wife," he says. But eating, he says, is different, more like height than morality in terms of its genetic influence.

"Currently, lean people think they stay lean because they are morally superior," O'Rahilly says. His work says it is because they are genetically lucky.

"I'm a big guy, and I'll never forget living with two thin people. I'm always struggling with my weight, and I cannot ever skip lunch because it makes me feel awful. They could come home and say, 'I didn't eat breakfast, and I forgot to eat lunch, and now I am absolutely starving.' Then they would go to the refrigerator and take out a few lettuce leaves and a few carrots and say, 'That was great. I feel so much better now.'"

O'Rahilly is saddened by the plight of his fat subjects and wants desperately to help them. "It is really bad to be morbidly obese. Not only is your life shortened, but your social life is miserable. No one wants to speak to you. You are socially isolated and poor because no one will employ you."

For now, he has nothing to offer most of his subjects, but he is working with drug companies who want to develop drugs that would, if they worked, treat his patients. The companies, of course, are hoping their drugs will work for obesity in general. O'Rahilly says his subjects are grateful that he is even asking the question of why they got so fat. "It helps hugely. They are really delighted that someone has taken them seriously. They had been told all along that they are just fat and lazy."

The dream is to do for the children with melanocortin-4 receptor deficiency and those with other defects along that pathway what he did for the girl who could not stop eating.

"What I believe is that we will be able to use the scientific understanding of appetite pathways to design treatments that will work for these severely obese people," O'Rahilly says.

"In that way," he insists, "we will prevail."

TEN MONTHS

If anyone had told Ron Krauss early on that he would hit his lowest weight ten months into the study and that the pounds he'd lost with such rigorous self-control would eventually slink back on, he would have been dubious. He had been doing so well for so long.

In January 2005, he weighed 190 pounds, nearly 50 pounds less than his starting weight of 237. His goal was to weigh 180, and he was close, so close. He bought new clothes and thought further weight loss was certain.

For months, he kept his weight steady, dropping sometimes as low as 185 before popping back up to 190, and for months he thought he might be in a lull before he dropped the remaining few pounds. The summer went by. "Then it started creeping back up," Ron says.

He blames himself.

"I got a little overconfident," he says. "My weight went up a few pounds, and I didn't pay a whole lot of attention." He stopped keeping records of what he was eating, he stopped keeping close watch over his portion sizes, and he found himself eating at night. "It's the ten o'clock cereal with banana. You say, 'It's not so bad.' But it's another 300 calories. You do that every day, and boom." Then there were the nights he had to work late. "I wasn't able to get out, so three Snickers bars were my dinner." Besides, Ron adds, "there's this reward mentality, particularly when things are very hectic and stressful; it's like food will make me feel better. It's like, 'Here, have some of this.'"

And those new clothes? He can't wear them anymore, Ron says. When he lost the weight, his friends all told him to throw away or give away those large clothes that hung like sacks on his body, but somehow he never did.

"That's when it really hit me. I had to start putting on my fat clothes," he says.

"The issue for me is maintaining the motivation to be disciplined," Ron continues. "It is one thing to know that a handful of peanuts is 190 calories. It is another thing not to eat it. I have this knowledge now. The question is, Do I choose to use it or not?"

Jerry Gordon reached his lowest weight six months into the study, when he'd lost 45 pounds. Then the weight loss stalled.

"I haven't lost any weight for, like, eight weeks," Jerry says. He is still exercising, he adds, working out on a StairMaster for half an hour a day, five days a week, and walking on a bike trail near his home. The problem, he explains, is "the eating. My calories are constantly inching up."

It is getting harder and harder for him to write down what he's been eating, to stick to the diet, he says. And it's not that he doesn't care.

"You reach a plateau, and then it's really, really tough," he says. "Let's say you plateau and you go three weeks where you still look at it like you're denying yourself. And you're denying yourself for no benefit. Then you say, 'You know what, why continue to do this? I'm not getting anywhere.' Then you start to reward yourself."

But Jerry was far from his goal when he hit that plateau. "I still had plenty of weight to lose. That's what really, really disappoints me," he says. How could his weight loss have stalled so soon?

"It was a blow to gain that weight back, no question about it. But who can I blame but myself? I realize that my portions have increased. I know my caloric intake is up again, and I just look the other way. I only regret that I don't have the self-discipline. That's my one regret."

Graziella Mann reached her lowest weight at about the same time as Jerry Gordon reached his. She'd lost 19 pounds from her starting weight of 223.

Now, she says, her weight loss has come to an abrupt halt.

"My weight stayed the same," she says. And that has happened even though she has become a fanatic exerciser. "I exercise every day. I get up at six in the morning and go to the gym."

But, Graz says, she also is realizing that exercise alone is not going to do it for her. "Somehow I was under the impression that if I walked for thirty minutes and my heart rate was 111, I would burn fat. Apparently it's a myth."

That leaves actual dieting and eating less, and, like Jerry, Graz is struggling.

"This week I was ill, and I had a couple of days when my calorie count was very low, in the 900s. But all of a sudden, I got my appetite back, and so I was, like, at 2,200 calories."

She's determined to get back on track. "I went back to measuring," Graz says. "I pulled out my digital scale." She again began writing down everything she ate, and even bought a software program that calculates calories and grams of fat. The results, she says, were quite a surprise. "I realized that my fat percentage was high," Graz tells the group. "It was 40 percent. I have to cut out using real mayonnaise and use something else. I have a really hard time with stuff like that—low-calorie and low-fat."

Now, she says, she is rededicating herself to the program. She will keep her food diary. And she will make better choices.

"I'm going to try to decrease the amount of fat I eat," Graz says. "I'm going to change what I snack on; I'm going to eat raw vegetables instead of cookies or chips, even light chips."

As for Carmen Pirollo, he says he lost his iron will after about six months, that magical time when everyone seemed to be doing so well. That's when his weight hit its low point, at 225 pounds, down from his starting weight of 260.

Now he's been gaining again, and he's worried. The meetings help, but their effect wears off quicker and quicker these days.

"I walk out of here on Monday night, and on Tuesday and Wednesday and Thursday I'm writing everything down, making sure it's perfect," Carmen says. "And then Friday comes, and the following week." And the recording? "It wanes," he says.

Carmen wants to keep his carb count down, "but there are times when you have to eat," he explains. At night, for instance, when he goes to sleep. He eats dinner at six or seven, and he can't bear going to bed with a gnawing emptiness in his stomach. "If there's not something in there, I can't sleep," he says. Then again, if he's eaten his carbs for the day, he's not supposed to have carbs at night, much as he might want them.

"What it boils down to is, What are you going to do to stay motivated and lose?" Carmen says. "If I don't have a workable strategy, it's like, Well, next week I'll do better."

But Carmen, like the others, is not about to give up.

"I'm not discouraged, by any means," he insists.

Carmen knows that in trying to lose weight, he is fighting his inheritance, his genes. "I come from a very heavy Italian family. The only thing that is discouraging is that I see myself making very good food choices and not having any impact. It's not that you can't lose weight—we've done that. But then you go back to where your genetics tells you to be.

"Very thin people can't imagine it," he says. "They think you're packing it in. They think it's a choice to be fat—just eat less and exercise more. Get off your rear end. They think that is an absolute truth. But it's not like that. And when you think of all the stigmas in life, stigmas against fat people, stigmas against gay people, it's because they think it's a choice to be fat, to be gay."

He adds, "When I talk to my students, who are only twelve years old, I tell them, 'There was a world before you were born and there were things that we considered absolute truths. And then they weren't.'"

8

The Fat Wars

No one could have been more determined than the dieters in the Penn study. They committed themselves to a two-year program. They kept food diaries. They exercised. They worked on avoiding thoughts and feelings and situations that tempted them to eat. And yet, as happens to dieters time and time again, most ended up gaining back almost every pound so painfully lost.

It's not as if they did not really care whether they lost weight. They had their dream weights that would, if they ever achieved them, let them go out into the world without the shame of being judged for being fat. They also said that losing weight was not just a matter of vanity. They worried about their health.

But the one type of question they seldom asked about weight loss was why. Why is there such an obesity obsession? Is being overweight that big a threat to health? Is it even bad for you to have a few extra pounds? This is a time when Americans and people in other developed countries are healthier than ever. We get fewer chronic diseases, and those we do get occur later in life. Disability rates are plummeting. We live longer and longer. It hardly appears that the health of America or of other nations is deteriorating. And so why does society cling to a beauty ideal that is so thin that almost no one can achieve it? If most of America is in the "overweight or obese" category, why aren't those plumper body types acceptable, even admired? Why has the nation's growing girth become such a fixation?

In a way, it seems puzzling. People are told they have only themselves to blame if they are fat. Diet evangelists preach the self-blame message. There's Mike Huckabee, for example, elected governor of Arkansas in 1996, who lost 105 pounds over a period of two years. He's been making almost a second career out of proselytizing that anyone who really wants to can lose weight. He told *The New York Times Magazine,* "We tend to demonize industries, but it's my fault that I was overweight. No one ever forced me to go to McDonald's and order a triple cheeseburger or the largest fries they had, along with a milkshake."

In a sense, Huckabee is right—people do have some control. The research shows that individuals have a range of weights, often spanning as much as 20 or 30 pounds, that they can achieve and sustain. Being at the bottom of your range usually means constant vigilance; being at the top can mean throwing all caution to the wind. People often say they feel better and have more energy when they are near the bottom of their natural weight range, but that if they try to go much below it, they are like the formerly obese people from those studies long ago at Rockefeller University—they become obsessed with food, they are always hungry, they find themselves bingeing and gorging despite their best intentions, and the pounds come back.

But there is another facet to the issue of self-control and obesity. It involves the science that has shown more clearly than ever that most people have limited power over their weight. The research has identified brain pathways that determine how much we eat, and those pathways are just as powerful as brain pathways controlling blood pressure and heart rate. The research includes decades of studies that have consistently shown that very few people lose substantial amounts of weight and keep it off.

So why is it that the scientific truths about obesity are so often unknown or ignored by anti-obesity crusaders and by struggling dieters? Why is it that even obesity fighters like Huckabee either do not know what science has learned or choose to ignore or deny it? Why is it that the dream weights of most overweight people are so low that they are biologically excruciatingly difficult, if not impossible, to maintain?

These are the hardest questions, the "why" questions, the ones that ask about society and politics and people's hopes and dreams. They start with the question, Why obesity? Of all health risks, why is obesity at the top?

Suppose there was one threat to health that you could simply wipe out overnight. Which would you choose? The answer should be clear, medical authorities say. There's no room for discussion. It's cigarette smoking.

But smoking's time as a health crisis has come and gone, a victim of short attention spans and, more important, the enormous success of the litigation against tobacco companies. People still smoke, but now what you hear about is obesity. There is not even a question in most people's minds that this is the health issue of the day. It pops up everywhere as a subject of concern. In November 2005, the University of Michigan held a half-day panel discussion on the state of women's health reporting—*women's* health, not simply health. About five hundred people attended, and they were asked to submit questions in writing for the panelists. And there it was, in the pile of yellow slips of paper with questions written on them—the obesity question. With Americans so fat and growing fatter, why don't the media write more about this terrible health crisis and exhort people to eat less and exercise more? Of course, the obesity question was not related specifically to women's health, but no one pointed that out. Joanne Silberner, a health reporter for National Public Radio (NPR), noted that NPR's health reporters never stop talking about obesity. In fact, NPR now has a "dedicated obesity reporter," she said, someone whose sole job it is to report on obesity. Then Michigan's surgeon general, Kimberlydawn Wisdom, one of the panelists sitting on the podium, chimed in, saying that when the magazine *Men's Health* declared Detroit America's fattest city, that helped enormously in getting people to pay attention to her office's new program, Michigan Steps Up. The program describes itself as a "healthy lifestyles campaign" and lists its goals in the following order: "Move More. Eat Better. Don't Smoke." It's hard to argue with such admonitions, but why was smoking number three? And was anyone any thinner for being told to exercise and eat better? She didn't say.

In part, the alarms arise from a growing segment of society—consisting of entities as diverse as drug companies, weight loss centers, academics, and divisions in federal and local governments—that depends on people being worried about the risks of being overweight or obese. "There are economic and professional interests in promoting this issue as opposed to other health issues," says Abigail Saguy, a sociologist at the University of California at Los Angeles.

Jeff Friedman agreed. "A lot of the reasons that perceptions about obesity are slow to change is that there is a huge financial and personal interest on the part of many promoting the message that 'this is your fault.' That includes the diet industry and a subgroup of the, quote, scientific community whose careers are invested in the idea that you can implement a set of behavioral measures that can treat obesity."

This is not to say that individuals and organizations that make their living from obesity are disingenuous. But when your support, and your money, comes from making sure that the growing number of obese and overweight people is a major public health priority, there may be at least subtle pressures to emphasize the dire consequences of weight gain and the importance of losing weight, whether or not the science fully backs those claims. And it is certainly true that if obesity were cured tomorrow, legions of companies and individuals would be out of work. Just a quick perusal of the vast array of professionals whose entire careers are centered on a concern over excess weight shows the extent to which the obesity problem has become part and parcel of the economy and the national mindset.

There are scientists, for example, who have just one research subject—obesity. Places like the Center for Weight and Eating Disorders at the University of Pennsylvania, where the study comparing the Atkins diet with a low-calorie one is taking place, exist to conduct weight loss study after weight loss study. They've been doing so for years even though Gary Foster, who was the center's clinical director (he's now director of the Center for Obesity Research and Education at Temple University), admits that every study pretty much ends the same way. The participants lose some weight, and then most gain it back. They may get special diet foods or special support, with psychologists like Leslie Womble or trainee Eva Epstein counseling them. They may get an unusual diet, like one the center was recruiting for in 2005 as the federal study of Atkins versus low-calorie diets wound down. (It's a study sponsored by the almond industry: participants in one group have to eat almonds as part of their low-calorie diet.) But no matter how the diets are tweaked, no matter how much psychological support the dieters get, the results have been absolutely predictable. The participants may end up more knowledgeable about what they are eating and more aware of portion sizes and calories. They may start exercising and be healthier for it. But most never achieve the goal they had when they joined the study—permanent and substantial weight loss. Nonetheless, the research goes on; the studies are repeated again and again.

Going up a step in the meta-analysis of the obesity world, there are the academic centers that exist just to study the national policies and practices that might be leading to obesity. At Yale, for example, the same building that houses the Yale Center for Eating and Weight Disorders—Yale's version of Penn's eating disorders center—also houses the Rudd Center for Food Policy and Obesity, whose research is more politically motivated. Its director, Kelly Brownell, who also directs the eating disorders center, wants junk food like sodas and candy banned from schools and wants taxes on junk foods, saying that obesity is caused by a "toxic environment."

Along with the academics studying obesity treatments and obesity politics, there are the federal agencies that support them, devoting large chunks of their workforce to the obesity problem. The Centers for Disease Control and Prevention (CDC), chief among them, says obesity is among its top four priorities in protecting public health. It has put its scientists to work studying obesity statistics and giving grants, and has been so enthusiastic about its anti-obesity mission that its research at times appears more like public relations than serious science.

There was, for example, a CDC study that Julie Gerberding, the agency's director, proudly announced in 2005 during a press conference on obesity statistics. She proclaimed that the centers sent a team of specialists into West Virginia to study an outbreak of obesity the same way the CDC studies an outbreak of an infectious disease. West Virginia had asked the CDC for help, saying it was the third-fattest state in the nation, with 27.6 percent of its adults classified as obese compared with 20.4 percent in the nation as a whole. And the state was fourth in the nation for diabetes, with 10.2 percent of its inhabitants affected as compared with 6.4 percent among people in the rest of the country. West Virginia also was number one in the prevalence of high blood pressure, with 33.1 percent of its people having the condition, as compared with 25.8 percent of the population nationwide.

"We were looking at our data," explained Kerri Kennedy, the program manager at the West Virginia Physical Activity and Nutrition Program, and saw that "we are facing a severe health crisis."

But an outbreak of obesity, of course, is nothing like an outbreak of food poisoning or influenza. It's clear what causes food poisoning or the flu, and there are well-tested measures to deal with those diseases. Not so with obesity. And other than garnering publicity for the CDC's efforts to stem the growing girth of the nation, it is hard to see what such an investigation of an obesity outbreak could accomplish. The study was directly modeled on the CDC's procedures when it is informed of a disease outbreak. With food poisoning, for example, teams try to find the source. If it is a restaurant, they interrogate employees and trace the food to its suppliers. Kerri Kennedy described a similar sequence of steps in the probe of the obesity outbreak. Teams went to schools and asked about physical education programs and what sort of food was provided. Did students get "at least one or two appealing fruits and vegetables every day"? And "would you replace sour cream with low-fat sour cream?" They went to workplaces and asked whether the vending machines had 100 percent fruit juices and bottled water (that ignores, of course, the fact that there are at least as many calories in fruit juices as in sodas) and whether there were policies to encourage people to exercise. Could people get an extra 15 or 20 minutes added to their lunch break if they chose to walk? The teams also went to randomly selected grocery stores and restaurants, asking whether they offered fruits and vegetables and skim or 1 percent milk.

Daniel McGee, a professor of statistics at Florida State University who has analyzed obesity data, burst out laughing when he heard about the West Virginia study. "My God," he said, "what a strange thing to do. They'll find out what we all know—that the country is no longer set up for physical exercise and that schoolchildren don't get a nutritious diet." And they'll find that "there is a lot of high-fat food on the shelves of every supermarket." But that, he added, "doesn't tell you much. I'm sure skinny people go to those same restaurants. Skinny kids go to those same schools."

The CDC is hardly alone in paying for uninformative studies. Other agencies, like the Department of Agriculture, also do their part.

On October 3, 2005, the Rand Corporation sent out a press release on findings from an obesity study paid for by the Department of Agriculture. "These findings may help explain the growing obesity epidemic among children over the past 20 years," said Roland Sturm, a Rand senior economist and lead author of the study.

That sounds impressive, but what did the scientists actually find? Not much, it turns out. They looked at the presence of convenience stores and full-service restaurants and fast food restaurants and grocery stores to see if there was a correlation with the weights of young school-aged children. They found no effect, defying the hypothesis in the CDC's West Virginia study. But they did report one positive finding: the higher the price of fruits and vegetables in a region, the fatter the young school-aged children. As any statistician will tell you, a correlation is hardly cause and effect. There are so many factors that could make a difference. Yes, income is a factor. Poor children, and poor adults, are likely to be fatter. But there are complicating factors. For example, the researchers had no data on how many fruits and vegetables the children ate, so they could not say whether people ate fewer fruits and vegetables in places where these cost more or even whether those children who gained more weight ate fewer fruits and vegetables. Nor could they say whether poor children wanted fruits and vegetables but shunned them because they were too expensive. Also, the Department of Agriculture had said previously that fruits and vegetables were cheap enough that even poor families could afford them. But that's okay. It just means another study is needed, the Rand researchers say. "Our findings suggest the need for more research to determine what impact the higher prices may have on the consumption of fruits and vegetables among children," they noted in their press release.

Of course, every area of science and medicine has silly studies or results that are much less convincing than a press release would have you believe. And other areas of medicine, like cancer or heart disease, also support a vast network of doctors, medical centers, and purveyors of drugs and supplements. But obesity really *is* different. It is one of the only areas of medical and social science research where everyone knows what the results must be—that children and adults are fat and getting fatter—and where everyone knows that the studies must show that the nation is heading toward a medical disaster. And it is an area where a few key culprits, or causes, must emerge. It's the lack of physical education in schools. It's the general slothfulness of Americans, who would rather take an elevator up one flight of steps than walk. It's those gargantuan portion sizes. It's Big Food, which, like Big Tobacco, has managed to produce products that are positively addictive. It's people's lack of individual responsibility, their unwillingness to be accountable for their own health. Anyone who really wants to can eat less and exercise more, some commentators say.

"Everyone has a deeply held set of beliefs, a hypothesis about the cause of obesity," says Jeff Friedman. Yet, he and others say, there is little objective scientific support for any of them. No one disputes that people really are fatter today. But, notes David Williamson, an obesity researcher at the CDC, national data do not indicate that Americans are any less active than they used to be.

If it's not physical activity, then are we eating more, or eating more of the wrong kinds of foods? Not necessarily, says Friedman. "It looks like food intake per capita is declining. And it looks like there is a reduction in the fraction of calories coming from fat." Still, something has to have changed. Why are people fatter now than they used to be? "That's the sixty-four-thousand-dollar question," Friedman says. Others, including Jules Hirsch at Rockefeller University, agree. "I don't know, and no one else does, either," he says.

One problem with looking at national statistics, Hirsch notes, is that obese people really do not eat significantly more than the non-obese. It takes just a few hundred more calories a day to sustain a fat person than a thin one, and data on food consumption may not be sensitive enough to show that. As for physical activity, almost no one does enough to make much difference in their caloric needs, so that is not a good indicator, either. Hirsch wonders whether something else is at play, some factor no one has thought of. The human race is changing for some reason, and body weight is only part of it. We're taller, more intelligent—at least according to IQ tests—and heavier. "We're different creatures than we used to be," Hirsch says.

"We're different and we store more fat." This may be an effect of something subtle, like better nutrition early in life, or less disease early in life. In animal studies and in some studies of people, small and very subtle changes in pregnancy or infancy or infections in infancy or childhood can affect conditions like obesity or the age of onset of chronic diseases in adulthood.

One thing is clear, though, Hirsch says. The admonitions to eat less and exercise more are not making a discernable difference in the weight of Americans. And it is not for lack of publicity about how important it is to lose weight. "You can't possibly saturate the country with any more warnings," Hirsch says. "I don't think anyone can say, 'Gee, I don't know about this.'"

That, of course, does not keep anyone from admonishing the public. And there's a reason for that, says Eric Oliver, a political scientist at the University of Chicago who studied the obesity epidemic. Obesity, he says, has something in it for everyone. "If you are on the political right, obesity is indicative of moral failure," he says. "If you are on the left, it means rampaging global capitalism."

Obesity alarms have long been part of American life, but they have been ratcheted up lately, and not just because Americans are fatter. Some social scientists trace the new urgency to a surgeon general's report, introduced with great fanfare at a press conference held in 2001.

It had all the trappings of a major event. The news was how fat Americans had become—two-thirds were overweight or obese, and there were at least twice as many obese people as in 1980. That was grim, David Satcher, the surgeon general, announced. "Overweight and obesity may soon cause as much preventable disease and death as cigarette smoking." Tommy G. Thompson, who was then secretary of the Department of Health and Human Services, emphasized the gravity of the situation: "Overweight and obesity are among the most pressing new health challenges we face today."

The surgeon general's report, "A Call to Action to Prevent and Decrease Overweight and Obesity," raised simmering concerns to a new level, one that James Morone, a political science professor at

Brown University, terms "crisis and obsession." The timing and setting were right, he added. "The surgeon general was the great force
behind the anti-tobacco campaign. In 2001, the tobacco settlements
were in place. We'd gotten all the cultural mileage out of blaming
tobacco for our sins. The surgeon general's report gave us a new sin,
and it resonated, it had a sense of truth."

"The operative term," says Sander Gilman, a distinguished professor of liberal arts and sciences at Emory University, "is moral
panic. There are moments when certain things become the focus of
the society because they are believed to be . . . a danger to the society, and it is believed that if you focus on it you will be able to avoid
it or cure it." That, he says, is the setting for a moral panic.

The moral panic inevitably includes the plight of children, and
that is no accident, Abigail Saguy says. "If you can play the child card
or the youth card, you are more effective. People are worried about
their children, and if you can play up those fears, you will get more
mileage."

The obesity moral panic had a "cultural resonance," Saguy notes.
"People don't like fatness. They don't like it for aesthetic reasons,
and they don't like it for moral reasons. They think it's ugly, and
they associate it with overconsumption." She also cites the tobacco
movement as a source of inspiration for the anti-obesity movement,
saying it provided a model for what could be accomplished. "Things
we didn't think were possible before the anti-tobacco movement became possible afterward," she says. Companies could be held liable
for selling a product that is legal but unhealthy. Social pressures could
change the image of smoking from glamorous to pitiable or even
despicable.

At the same time, Saguy said, the moral panic over obesity played
into the decline of the welfare state and the increasing emphasis in
American society on personal responsibility. It introduced a socially
acceptable venue for demeaning the poor and, especially, black
women and Mexican-Americans, who are more likely than affluent
whites to be fat, she said. In fact, Saguy added, the very language
used to discuss obesity is illuminating. "Obesity is a health risk, like
smoking, rather than a physical trait, like race. You wouldn't ask
how risky it is to be black, although you would ask whether blacks

have a greater tendency to certain illnesses. The risk frame implies that obesity is under people's control. It assumes that people are to blame for their weight."

But one of the great ironies of the moral panic over obesity is that when scientists have conducted rigorous federally funded studies that cast doubt on some of the most basic assumptions about the dangers of being overweight and what to do about it, their results have been ignored or attacked as the moral panic goes on.

Two large studies in the 1990s, for example, asked whether the measures usually advocated to prevent children from gaining weight are effective. One was an eight-year, $20 million project sponsored by the National Heart, Lung, and Blood Institute (part of the National Institutes of Health). It followed 1,704 third graders in forty-one elementary schools in the Southwest, chosen because their students were mostly Native Americans and at great risk for obesity. The schools were randomly assigned to be left alone or to be the subjects of an intensive intervention, and the question that was asked was whether, by grade 5, the children in the intervention schools would be thinner than those in the schools that served as controls.

The study's principal investigator was a highly regarded scientist, Benjamin Caballero, director of the Center for Nutrition at Johns Hopkins University's Bloomberg School of Public Health. He explains the study design: If a school was assigned to the special intervention program, the food served there would be changed to make it healthy and low-fat and teachers would regularly instruct the children on how to choose the most nutritious and least fattening foods. These low-income children ate both breakfast and lunch at school, Caballero says, and food eaten at school supplied half of their calories each day. The researchers also included the children's families in the study, bringing them to the schools every month or every other month for special events. In addition, the children often prepared healthy snacks at school and would take a lunchbox home, showing what sort of food they should be eating. Then, Caballero said, "the parents would come to the schools, and the children would cook for the parents." As for physical activity, the researchers made sure that the children had an hour of real physical exertion at least three times a week—the goal was to have an hour a day of exercise. That meant going beyond the usual physical education classes, he explained. "We created this thing called exercise breaks in which the teacher had to stop the class, turn on the music," and, he said, the children danced. The breaks occurred at least two and sometimes three times a day, every day.

And the results? The children in the schools that had the special programs learned their lessons well. They could recite chapter and verse on the importance of activity and proper nutrition. They also ate less fat. At the start, their diet was about 34 percent fat; at the end, after two years of the program, it was 27 percent fat. But alas, Caballero said, "it was not enough to change body weight."

He published his paper in the *American Journal of Clinical Nutrition* in 2003 to an absolute silence. No press release, no media coverage, no invitations to speak about the results at scientific meetings. And here's the indicator that was perhaps most surprising: the *American Journal of Clinical Nutrition*, like other medical journals, lists on its Web page links to other articles that have referenced this one. The number of times anyone referenced Caballero's obesity article? Zero. When asked about that in an e-mail, Caballero replied: "You are very perceptive, my friend. The study continues to be essentially ignored in the U.S., in spite of being the only one so far of its kind, $20 million over 8 years, extremely rigorous data collection, etc."

But the intervention's failure to affect the children's weight was a puzzle. If such methods worked at all, you might expect them to work among Native American children, who have a very high risk of becoming obese. Usually, when scientists conduct clinical trials, they deliberately study groups that are likely to have the condition under study—they will test a method they hope will prevent heart disease in a study of smokers or people with high blood pressure and high cholesterol levels. A prevention for diabetes will be tested among those whose blood sugar is starting to climb. The reason is that if the group is prone to develop the condition you are interested in, there will be more people who do get that condition over the course of the study, giving you greater statistical power to see if the intervention works. So a group of children at high risk for growing fat seemed like the perfect study subjects. But maybe the problem was that they were at *such* high risk that these simple measures were inadequate. Maybe if you provided the same interventions to children at average risk for obesity, the results would be very different.

Unfortunately, as another large, and ignored, study found, that is not the case.

The other study also was sponsored by the National Institutes of Health and also involved third graders who were given interventions until fifth grade, and it also had a three-year follow-up to see if the children in the intervention group learned their lessons. It included 5,106 children from ninety-six schools in California, Louisiana, Michigan, and Texas. Fifty-six schools were randomly assigned to have the intervention—healthy food, nutrition instruction, extra physical activity—and forty schools served as controls. The study's researchers describe it as "the largest school-based randomized trial ever conducted."

The researchers reported their results in a paper published in 1999 in the *Archives of Pediatrics and Adolescent Medicine*. It turned out that the children in the schools with the special programs learned their lessons, and their diet-recall questionnaires indicated that they ate less fat. They also exercised more. And they retained their knowledge for years afterward. But their weights were no different from those of children in the schools that served as controls.

Perhaps it should have come as no surprise. After all, Mickey Stunkard concluded in the 1980s that the children who are going to get fat are those whose biological parents are fat, and that applies to adopted children as well as children living with their biological parents. But his message, too, was largely ignored, and today school systems are banning sodas and changing the food in cafeterias to combat obesity. They are adding physical education and even putting pedometers on children to keep track of how many steps they take. That may be fine; the children may be healthier or happier, but the promise is that this is going to prevent them from getting fat.

Even the National Institutes of Health, which sponsored the two large studies on children, is acting as though the studies never existed, starting a new program called "We Can" to involve parents and schools in changing children's diet and adding more exercise into their day. It's not a study—perhaps the day of large studies asking whether interventions helped is over. Instead, it is a way of putting those interventions into action, with or without evidence that they work. The National Institutes of Health describes "We Can" as "a national program designed as a one-stop resource for parents and caregivers interested in practical tools to help children 8–13 years old stay at a healthy weight. Tips and fun activities focus on *three* critical behaviors: *improved* food choices, *increased* physical activity and *reduced* screen time."

Caballero says he understands why the rigorous science has been ignored. People are alarmed about obesity in children, and what can you tell them? That nothing has been shown to prevent it? "There is some social pressure to do something," he says. So, he says, rather than cite the two large studies, "people go back to smaller studies" that, although they are too small or poorly designed to prove anything, provide hints that, maybe, the interventions work.

And both he and Philip R. Nader, who directed the study of ninety-six schools and is an emeritus research professor at the University of California at San Diego, think they know why their studies failed—the intervention was not enough. It is necessary to change the children's total experience, not just what happens at school. "Not only the school, but the family, the community, the grocery store," Caballero said.

That, of course, remains to be demonstrated, although the lack of evidence has not prevented people from advocating changes in the entire environment. Ban advertising of junk foods. Build more sidewalks. The list goes on. It reminds one scientist, David Freedman, a statistician at the University of California at Berkeley, of what he sees as people's "wonderful capacity for ignoring negative evidence." If studies failed to find that changing the environment in schools makes any difference, then the popular solution, it seems, is not to question the premise but rather to increase the intensity of the intervention.

Freedman, who has written books on the science and history of clinical trials, recalls a story about a nineteenth-century French doctor who was a pioneer in the medical application of statistics, Pierre-Charles-Alexandre Louis. Louis did a study on the effect of bloodletting, or bleeding, on pneumonia. Bloodletting was the standard treatment at the time, and so Louis was astonished when his study showed it didn't work. "Dr. Louis rejected this as terrifying and absurd," Freedman says. So he made a recommendation: Bleed earlier and bleed harder.

But ignoring or explaining away inconvenient findings is just one response. The other is to attack them. That is what happened to a group of scientists who asked a fundamental question: How dangerous is it to your health to be overweight?

They began, they say, because they saw a meaty statistical problem that they had not considered before, and because they are statisticians and epidemiologists, such challenges are their passion. The question was, How many Americans die each year simply because they are so fat?

The answer is not easy to decide, the researchers realized, because they had to take into account everything other than obesity that could lead to death—smoking, age, chronic diseases—and then ask what was left for obesity's contribution. That meant not only devising statistical methods, but also getting reliable national data. So two of the scientists, Katherine Flegal, a statistician at the National Center for Health Statistics, and David Williamson, an epidemiologist at the CDC, set to work.

Shortly after they began, one of their colleagues, David Allison of the CDC, published his own attempt to answer the question. His paper, which appeared in 1999 in the *Journal of the American Medical Association*, was startling. It claimed that 280,000 to 350,000 Americans die each year because they weigh too much. This was the first time anyone had published a paper that made a serious, rigorous attempt to estimate obesity's death toll, and as expected, the paper elicited cries of alarm and hand-wringing.

But when Flegal and Williamson read that paper, they suspected that Allison's statistical methods were not correct. He had used data from six studies that followed a general pattern. Scientists weighed people or, more often, asked them what they weighed, and then checked back a decade later to see if their subjects were dead or alive. "Then you use a statistical model that tries to relate the increase in the death rate in obese subjects to the death rate in people who are what you decide is the normal weight," Williamson said. But this is not as straightforward as it sounds, because there are other factors, such as age, sex, and smoking habits, that might affect survival, and these same factors might affect weight. Statisticians have to correct for these confounding factors, a difficult task.

And that was the problem with Allison's paper in his view, Williamson says. "To our knowledge, David Allison was the first person who took the relative risk—the rate of death in obese people related to the rate of death in this reference group of normal weight. David Allison did that and he was a pioneer," Williamson said. "But Katherine had read his paper very carefully, and she called me one day and said, 'Have you read his paper recently?' I said no, and she said, 'Take a look at the following issues.'" Her questions were sophisticated and had slipped by many scientists, but they cast serious doubt on the paper's conclusions. In essence, Williamson explains, when Allison made his calculations of the number of deaths attributable to obesity, he assumed that the data had not already taken into account factors, like smoking, that can independently alter the death rate. But, in fact, they had been adjusted for such factors. The result, Williamson and Flegal decided, was that the statistics could overestimate the number of deaths caused by obesity by 15 or 20 percent. They decided to publish a paper showing the error.

"We were trying to figure out methods, and we wrote a theoretical paper showing how age and causes of death could make a difference," Flegal says. "It took four years to get it published. We sent it to four journals, and they returned it without reviewing it." Finally, it appeared in the *American Journal of Public Health*.

But, Flegal confesses, while she and Williamson convinced themselves that the other scientists were getting the statistics wrong, they still were not sure how to get them right. "We were flailing around," she says. And there was another problem. If you want to know the number of deaths caused by obesity, you should have a representative sample of the U.S. population. Allison had not had that. He'd used data from studies, such as a major long-term Harvard study of nurses, that consisted of people who were better educated and more health-conscious than most people. Those studies also tended to selectively remove people from their populations, excluding large numbers of nurses in the nurses' study, for example, because the researchers thought they were sick. Such practices have become increasingly common in studies of obesity, although they are rarely seen elsewhere in epidemiology because there is no agreed-upon way to decide whom to remove, or when, and such a practice inevitably alters the results. "I think it's a very questionable approach," Williamson says.

But it is one thing to say why you think someone else is wrong. It is another to do the study in a way that corrects for those errors and gets the statistics right. Flegal and Williamson asked two experienced scientists at the National Cancer Institute to help them. The statisticians, Barry Graubard and Mitchell Gail, were new to the obesity field, but they had developed highly regarded and sophisticated methods for estimating cancer risks and were intrigued by the obesity problem. The statistical challenge was the same as with cancer, and their experience with national cancer data could carry over, they decided.

Finally, the group of researchers got what they thought were reliable methods and national data from the federal National Health and Nutritional Examination Survey. The result was what they considered to be accurate estimates of obesity's death toll. And, to their own surprise, the researchers found that that toll was not nearly as bad as the earlier studies had indicated.

One reason for their lower estimate, the group decided, was the source of their data. That national survey gave them a representative sample of the U.S. population, as well as data they could trust on heights and weights. In the survey, people were actually weighed and measured, not just asked their height and weight.

The scientists knew what they had found was important to the obesity debate. If you accepted their methods and their data, you could no longer say that hundreds of thousands of Americans were dying each year because, quite frankly, they were too fat. Their study said that rather than being at an increased risk of death, overweight people were, if anything, better off. Their death rate was slightly lower than the death rate for so-called normal-weight people. The mortality curves were U-shaped, with increased risks of death at both ends, the very thin and the very obese. The implication was that, as far as mortality was concerned, overweight was the best weight to be.

In the meantime, the *Journal of the American Medical Association* published another paper, by different researchers from the CDC and

necessarily even representative of their own study populations. The same held for the data from the American Cancer Society, he said. The reason is that both studies excluded most of their subjects from their analysis, deciding that they should not be counted because they were sick, or because they were smokers, or for some other reason; one analysis of the nurses' study excluded nearly 90 percent of the deaths. "We have data sets that are truly nationally representative of the U.S. population," Williamson said. And, Flegal noted, their group used actual measured weights and heights, not self-reported ones as were used by the Harvard and the American Cancer Society investigators. That means Flegal's group probably had more accurate numbers, since people notoriously claim that they weigh less than they really do.

As for their statistical methods, Flegal says, she and her colleagues had analyzed their data in a variety of ways. They looked at the results both with and without current or former smokers and people who had chronic diseases. They posted the extensive analysis on the Internet—journals like the *Journal of the American Medical Association* allow for only so much additional data—and the results always came out the same: There was no mortality risk from being overweight and little from being obese, with the exception of the extremely obese, whose death risk was slightly higher.

Barry Graubard said he was used to cancer epidemiology and statistics, in which scientific disagreements are usually resolved by discussion and careful consideration of the data. He had just not appreciated the strong feelings people have when anyone questions whether being overweight is really bad for your health.

"This whole thing is a really strange mix of politics, science, and the personal way people view themselves and their condition," he says. "And there's an economic aspect, too. It's a very volatile mix of all these things. I think our paper was almost like a lens on this issue. It brought out the worst in everyone. I have never seen anything like this before. I was stunned by the whole reaction."

Flegal said she was stunned. Harvard researchers holding a *seminar* to refute her? It was unheard of in the nominally polite world of science. "I don't know what to say. I don't have a problem with people at a conference talking about their data, but I do have a problem with their talking about our data and saying we should have found the same things that they found." And why, she asked, were people so upset with her findings? "Isn't this good news? Isn't it good that people are not dying?"

Even the group's credentials came under attack, Williamson said. "Some went after us individually, which is okay, but it doesn't really advance public understanding. Some attacked our credentials because we are not physicians. Katherine and I have Ph.D.'s in human nutrition, but one of the people who criticized our credentials is the head of a department of nutrition. Hopefully, he thinks nutrition is an important field." Mitchell Gail, Williamson added, got his M.D. degree from Harvard and also has a Ph.D. in statistics, as does Barry Graubard. "I've published papers with most of our critics, and our credentials didn't seem to be an issue then," Williamson says.

But that was not the end of it. Soon, the Harvard group issued a press release with a single message: Americans were not persuaded by the study done by Flegal, Williamson, Graubard, and Mitchell. The release, sent to reporters by e-mail on July 14, 2005, stated:

> The past year has seen scientific studies that have varied in their estimates of the seriousness of obesity and overweight and their impact on premature death. A new opinion poll by the Harvard School of Public Health finds that most Americans have not changed their minds about the seriousness of the obesity problem and do not believe that scientific experts are overestimating the health risks of obesity. In addition, they are no less likely than a year ago to be keeping track of calories, fat content, or the amount of carbohydrates they eat.

It added that many people believe being overweight is as bad as smoking: "Forty-one percent of Americans reported believing that the same number of people in the US die from the effects of being seriously overweight as from the effects of smoking and tobacco." And about half thought someone who was even moderately overweight was likely to die prematurely, despite the finding by Flegal, Williamson, Graubard, and Gail that this is not so and that, in fact, the death rate was lowest among the overweight.

Obesity researchers wrote editorials and letters urging action to combat the paper. James O. Hill of the University of Colorado, one of the principal investigators in the study comparing the Atkins diet with a low-calorie one, editorialized to doctors in the journal *Obesity Management*, where he is editor in chief. Writing in the June 2005 issue, he said,

> Your patients likely did not read the original article, but they did likely hear about it in the news and the message they got was not to worry so much about overweight and obesity. I do not think this is the message you want them to have. It is difficult enough to get many people interested in addressing their excessive weight. Second, when we need more resources not just to study obesity but to begin to do something about it for the public, this provides ammunition for those who oppose this allocation of resources.

He called on doctors to get involved: "I would like to challenge you to write a letter to your local newspaper stating your view and giving your firsthand impressions of overweight and obesity. We especially need to hear from pediatricians who are seeing more and more overweight children."

Flegal says she had a real education in the politics of obesity.

"Everyone thinks they already know the answer," she says. "Anything that doesn't fit, they have to explain it away or ignore it. All these people who just know weight loss is good for you. It's just taken for granted regardless of the evidence." She was not naïve about her findings, she said. "I expected people would get perturbed, but I really didn't expect the way they did it. All these erroneous so-called fact sheets. And these misinterpretations and making up things we'd said."

She saw the prevailing attitude in action: "It seems like some researchers say to themselves, 'If the data don't come out as strongly as we want, then let's just work on these data until they come out the way we want them to.'"

Oddly enough, that disputed paper by Flegal and her colleagues was hardly the only evidence that the healthiest weights are the ones deemed overweight. There also is another line of research that is seldom mentioned by obesity researchers, perhaps because it involves papers published in economics journals and because the papers are about health, not obesity. The work began in the 1980s when Robert Fogel, a Nobel laureate in economics at the University of Chicago Graduate School of Business, began a daunting task—to examine the records of 45,300 Union Army soldiers to see how tall people were in those days. The idea was that adult height is an indicator of general health and nutrition, and he wanted to compare the men at the time of the Civil War with the men of more recent generations.

The project grew and came to encompass medical records and census records and to include studies of Europeans, including Norwegians, the French, and the British, as well as people in less-developed nations, like Ghana.

The work is still continuing, but over and over again, Fogel and his many colleagues find that as populations grew healthier, as happened in America and Europe, they grew taller and fatter. When the researchers drew graphs of heights and weights and health—including the incidence of chronic diseases and death rates—they saw a consistent pattern. The graphs were shaped like U's, with higher death rates at the lowest and highest body mass indexes. It is not clear why that would happen, but it occurs in every population that has been studied. And the best weights for health consistently included ones in the overweight range.

Could that mean that the obesity epidemic is actually a good thing, with heights increasing because of better nutrition and freedom from disease, and with weights increasing, too, to allow the average person the best possible health?

"We don't know that yet," Fogel says. "It's a reasonable hypothesis, but a lot of this is playing your hunches. I tend to be, 'Well, maybe.' I certainly would not forecast it on the basis of what I know, but I also would not rule it out."

Underlying the debate on the health risks of being overweight were two basic assumptions: If you are fat, you can lose weight and keep it off if you really want to. And if you do lose weight, you are then as healthy as someone who was never fat. But, asks Barry Graubard, how do you know that a formerly fat person has the same health risks as someone the same weight who is naturally thin?

"That's what bothers me," he says. "Weight is not an exposure; it's an outcome. It's not like smoking—you can smoke or not, and it's clear that tobacco causes illness" and stopping smoking reduces that risk. "It's not clear if losing weight makes a difference in disease." The problem is getting data, finding people who voluntarily lost weight and kept it off and asking whether their health was different when they were thinner. And the reason that is a problem is that there are very few people who have lost substantial amounts of weight and kept it off. In fact, the only method that routinely leads to long-term weight loss for most people is surgery. And the one study so far that rigorously assessed health after surgery did not quite find what many in the obesity field assume to be true.

The study, which took place in Sweden, involved about twelve hundred people who weighed an average of about 250 pounds. Half had stomach-reducing bariatric surgery, and the rest tried on their own, unsuccessfully as it turned out, to lose weight. The question was, What happened to the blood pressure, cholesterol levels, and blood sugar levels of the surgery patients as compared with those of people who remained fat? The surgery patients had less diabetes—ten years after the study began, 13 percent of those who had surgery had diabetes as compared with 36 percent of those who did not have the operation. But blood pressure and cholesterol were a different story. For the first year, they looked good. The surgery patients saw their cholesterol levels and blood pressures drop. But then they began rising again, drifting up to levels that were slightly higher than before the operation. Within two years after the operation, any beneficial blood pressure and cholesterol effects were gone.

Supporting the observations from the surgery study is another study that also calls into question the notion that getting rid of extra fat will result in a permanent decline in cholesterol and blood pressure levels.

This study was conducted by plastic surgeons who wanted health insurance to pay for liposuction. Their idea was that if they could remove about 20 pounds of abdominal fat from obese women, they would see improvements in cholesterol levels, blood pressure, and blood sugar. That would imply a health benefit. It was an unusually large amount of fat to remove, but the plastic surgeons wanted to remove as much as dieters can expect to lose with the most advanced diet and weight loss drug regimens—about 12 percent of their body fat—reasoning that that should be enough to make a real difference in health.

The study, published in the *New England Journal of Medicine* in 2004, found no such thing.

The women were thinner after liposuction, and they no longer had so much abdominal fat, but nothing else changed. The question was, Why? One possibility, the investigators wrote, was that diets may be eliciting beneficial effects not because people weigh less, but rather because the process of losing weight itself causes cholesterol, blood sugar, and blood pressure levels to drop. This makes sense, they add, because when people diet, these metabolic measures start to improve immediately, within days, and long before the dieters have lost any fat. With the liposuction, though, the pounds were gone instantly, without the metabolic change that comes from eating less food than the body requires, a change that forces the body to burn its own fat for fuel.

"Our results suggest that induction of a negative energy balance, not simply a decrease in the mass of adipose tissue, is critical for achieving the metabolic benefits of weight loss," the authors wrote. "Even small amounts of weight loss induced by a negative energy balance affects many variables pertaining to body-fat composition and lipid metabolism—variables that probably contribute to the metabolic abnormalities associated with obesity."

Another possibility, they add, is that maybe liposuction removes the wrong *kind* of fat. Maybe fat deeper down in the body is the kind you want to remove, and that is beyond the reach of liposuction. There was no way of testing that idea, of course, but they did fail to confirm their hypothesis that simply getting rid of 20 pounds of fat will improve health.

So if you are fat but not diabetic, if you're basically a healthy fat person, should you lose weight for medical reasons? Jeff Friedman says the answer is unknown. "If you are obese and don't have comorbidities [other medical problems], what is the health benefit of weight loss? I don't think we know that at all," Friedman says.

Then why lose weight? For many, health is only part of the issue. It goes back to Carmen Pirollo's observation: "I'm an American. We live in a society where people have to be beautiful."

TWO YEARS

The two diet groups have their last meeting on a breezy Monday evening, March 6, 2006. It would be their last time to enter the grimly utilitarian office building on Market Street in Philadelphia, the last time to take the elevator to the third floor, get off, walk through a set of glass doors, turn left, and walk down a narrow corridor to the bleak room where the groups have been meeting for the past two years. They might be expecting that it will be a time to reassess what those two years have been like. It will be a moment of truth. Whether or not they lost much weight, the experience has been one of those rare events that change someone as a human being. They are leaving the study fundamentally different from the way they were when they arrived.

But most of the dieters do not show up. Perhaps some are too busy, or perhaps the real truth is that they are too disheartened. They've seen a lot in the past two years. They started with such high hopes, such optimistic dreams, and now reality has set in. And the exciting battle of the diets that drew them to the study in the first place is seeming tired and worn. Everyone had wanted the Atkins diet when they signed up. Now, two years later, few would ever choose it. As quickly as it began, the Atkins diet fad crested and that weight loss scheme lost its allure. On August 1, 2005, Atkins Nutritionals, the company that Robert Atkins, the diet guru, founded in 1989, filed for bankruptcy. Companies were jettisoning low-carb products, looking for the next new thing. Whole grains, some companies decided. Low-sugar. No trans fats.

One man in the Atkins group calls the diet he's been on for two years "this goofy Atkins diet."

Carmen Pirollo comes to that last meeting, but some bitterness has been creeping into his voice of late. He says he understands now just what he has gotten into. "They finally told us. They put it point blank," he says. "They told us, 'This really wasn't for you to lose weight. It was for us to get data to see what worked and what didn't. You're really guinea pigs, and if you get something out of it, fine.' If not, they are still looking for hard data.

"We were there the whole two years," Carmen says. "We've been even more involved in the study than the people who were running it. We lost Brooke [a study coordinator]. We haven't seen Leslie for a number of months," he adds, referring to Leslie Womble, who has not come to many meetings since the birth of her second daughter in 2005. "We all know this is for a doctoral dissertation for Eva," Carmen continues, referring to Eva Epstein, who was using her work with the groups to fulfill requirements for a Ph.D. in clinical psychology from Temple University. "When you don't see the people who are supposed to be there to support you, when it's not important to them, it's not important to you, either."

At that last meeting, Eva (who is there without Leslie, who is out of town, Eva says) announces that the Penn study director, Gary Foster, is moving to Temple University and his part of the study will move with him. The dieters have to fill out new consent forms giving their data to Temple.

The dieters ask Eva when they will finally learn the results of the study. She does not know, she tells them, advising them to just keep watching, since surely the study will make the news when it is finally completed, analyzed, and published. It is clear from her response, though, that there are no plans to keep the dieters in the loop.

As parting gifts, she gives them each a T-shirt, size extra-extra-large, and a University of Pennsylvania mug.

Yet in March 2006, the diet study is far from complete. At Penn, a diet group like theirs started just a year ago and still had a year left. And even when all the groups at all three medical centers finish their two years of dieting, the data have to be analyzed, a paper has to be written, all the coauthors have to sign off on it, the paper has to be sent to a medical journal for review, and finally, once the paper is accepted, it could be months before it is published. At that point, the question might be, Will the results really matter? In an inadvertent way, it turns out that the question being asked in the Atkins-versus-low-calorie study was answered by another, much larger study, published in early 2006.

That was a study sponsored by the Women's Health Initiative of the National Institutes of Health, and its question was whether a low-fat diet could prevent breast cancer. The nearly forty-nine thousand women who participated were randomly assigned to follow a low-fat diet or their normal diet for eight years. It was, in a way, a reverse Atkins study. If Atkins was right that what really matters is *what* you eat, not *how much* you eat, if he was right that carbohydrates make you fat and give you diabetes and high cholesterol levels, then the women following the low-fat diet, who were eating many more carbohydrates, should have gotten fatter and suffered health problems. They did not. At the end of the study, the low-fat and the regular-diet women weighed the same and there were no differences in health between the two diet groups. Nor were there differences in markers of health, including blood sugar and cholesterol levels.

Yet all the Penn study participants, even those who did not come to that last meeting, say they have changed because they joined the study and the change was for the good.

"I think we all agree it's been a fascinating two years, an almost transforming two years," says a man in the Atkins group. "I lost weight; I gained some of it back. I think I have a good idea of what I can realistically accomplish, which is a lot different than what I thought two years ago. I went through this thing, What's your dream weight? I think I'm more realistic now."

Eating without thinking—that had been her habit, says Graziella Mann. But no more. She remembers those days two years earlier when she was accepted into the study and told to keep a food diary for a month before the diet began.

"They said, 'All we want you to do is write down what you eat and when you eat it. Eat naturally. Just tell us what you eat.' So I did. The first day I wrote two pages of items. I looked at it and said,

'Oh my God.' By the third day, it was a really short list. I had been made aware that I was eating all day long. It might have been something small, a bar of chocolate, but I was always eating." Astonished, she self-consciously stopped much of her constant grazing. "Between that time and the time the program started, I lost 10 pounds."

Now, Graz says, she can't imagine eating so reflexively and her food choices have changed. She used to start her day by going to a convenience store and getting doughnuts and coffee, liberally pouring in cream. "I don't eat doughnuts anymore," she says. "I know if I make that choice to go to Wawa every morning and get doughnuts and get the coffee with all the cream, I know where that's going to take me. I know there are better choices. I pick organic things; I pick natural things; I pick low-fat things. I don't pick them because I have to. It's what I like eating now. It's become a part of me. This is not really a diet. It's a way of life."

She also exercises regularly, something she had never done before, and she sees the effects every day. "I feel much better. I can run for a train now and not get winded."

And her weight? She's come to terms with it, Graz says, and she knows that for people like her, who have been fat all their lives, it is just not realistic to expect to become truly thin and stay there. "We're not going to lose the 50 to 100 pounds. I may not be that poster child for dieting, but I am very happy. I am still 212 pounds, down from 223 when I first signed up, but I'm much healthier. And why *can't* a woman be 212 pounds?"

Jerry Gordon is a changed person, too. He knows portion sizes; he reflexively estimates the calories in every bit of food he sees. "You start thinking in terms of portions," he says, something he never did before. And he exercises regularly, walking and using the StairMaster he has at his house. "It sets a certain tone for a healthy lifestyle," he says. "It makes a big difference in your attitude if you can say, 'I'm exercising every day and maintaining some kind of control and discipline.'"

Jerry remains fat. "Will I ever reach a normal weight? No," he says. "That's not going to happen. But I'd say I'm definitely happier."

As for Carmen, his story is much the same as the others'. He is acutely aware of everything he eats, but he is still obese. "I guess we

all are," he says. "I had a goal and I reached it, and now I'm growing again." But he says, "They told us not to think of ourselves as
failures and I don't."

Ron Krauss knows calorie counts so well that even when he decides to eat more than he thinks he should, he's tallying up the calories
in his head. He's learned to control his environment by keeping foods
he can't resist, like ice cream, out of his house. "If it's there, I'll eat
it," he says. But he, too, is not thin.

"I ended up, if I don't gain any more weight, about 30 pounds
lighter. I lost about 15 percent of my body weight. And I do feel better about myself in general," he says. "I sort of think the real effect of
this program, at least for me, won't become evident at least for another year or so when I see if I can lose some of the weight I've put
back on and maintain it."

A week later, he sends an e-mail saying he's on his way. "I've just
gone back to the basics of the program, keeping a record of what
I'm eating and trying to keep in the 1800/2000 calorie range," he
writes. And he's lost 2 pounds and invented a breakfast he loves—
he mixes one of those packets of instant oatmeal into a cup of yogurt.
"Besides adding flavor and texture, the oatmeal adds protein, fiber,
and low-glycemic carbs, and only about 120 calories."

In the end, though, the lesson is, once again, that no matter what the
diet and no matter how hard they try, most people will not be able
to lose a lot of weight and keep it off. They can lose a lot of weight
and keep it off briefly, they can lose some weight and keep it off for
a longer time, they can learn to control their eating, and they can
learn the joy of regular exercise. Those who do best tend to be those
who learn to gauge portions and calories and to keep their houses
as free as possible of food they cannot resist. The effort, the *lifelong*
effort, can be rewarding—people say they feel much better for it.
But true thinness is likely to elude them.

And that, says Carmen, is a bittersweet lesson.

He believed that wanting to be thin was most of the battle. Now,
looking back, he knows that is not enough.

"There were millions of people out there who turned to phen-fen or anything they could. If weight loss would just come in a wish, everyone would be thin."

He used to think that he would find the perfect diet, would lose all the weight he wanted to lose, and then would keep it off. Now, he says, he realizes that he does not really have that kind of control over what he eats.

"In your brain, you say, 'I've got 100 percent free will. I have total control over what I eat.' But in the experience of my life, in the experience of my day, in the experiences that have been thrust upon me, I don't have that control."

He used to believe that this diet would be the last—it was going to work, and he would never be fat again.

Now he knows that cannot happen. He's not ready to diet again just yet, but he knows that day will come.

"There are those moments when you say, 'I couldn't go on a diet now for love or money.' And there are those times when you say, 'Now's the time. I'm going to do it again.' I probably will be one of those people who diet for the rest of their lives. Or let's not call it dieting. Let's call it monitoring. I will be monitoring my weight for the rest of my life."

But don't pity him, Carmen says.

"You know, weight isn't the worst thing in the world. Thank God, I just have to monitor my weight. That's the least of my problems."

Epilogue

I t was a transforming two years for the dieters. And it was a transforming time for me, too, making me wonder about the seductive power of dieting and its siren call.

I told a skinny acquaintance about the Penn dieters I had been following and the sad, but predictable, outcome of their attempts to lose weight. "Did they really, really try?" he asked. I drew in my breath. It was like a slap. "Yes, *of course* they really, really tried," I said. Of course, of course. How could they have tried any harder? I thought of Jerry Gordon, playing cards with his friends who were laughing and snorting, saying he felt like the librarian because he turned down the drinks, turned down the food. I thought of Carmen Pirollo, taking his Atkins snacks when he went to the movies with his friend, telling himself that the smell of popcorn was not even tempting. I thought of Graziella Mann, hiring a personal trainer, going to the gym at 6:00 a.m. I thought of two years of the study and all the effort and the eternal hope of those dieters, the trying again and the rededicating themselves and the getting back to those food diaries. *Of course* they really, really tried.

But perhaps that thin man's question should be no surprise. Who could miss the drumbeat of messages from scientists and weight loss experts, the incessant hectoring year in and year out, assuring fat people that everything is possible for those who really, really try. Yes, you can lose weight and keep it off, and yes, it is important, crucially important, to try and try again to diet, no matter how often you have failed. And yes, you do need to be educated about what foods to eat, and companies do need to be pressured to sell healthier foods.

While I was working on this book, I interviewed a psychologist, Peter Herman of the University of Toronto, who studies the psychology of false hope. Dieting is the exemplar, he told me. At first, he thought it made no sense to try one diet after another the way Carmen did, the way most of the others in the Penn group did, the way most fat people do. Why, Herman asked, do people keep trying to lose weight, going on diet after diet, when they are let down time and time again? "If psychology ever taught us anything, it's that if you fail to reinforce a behavior, it should extinguish," he said. Why is dieting the exception?

"You have to ask yourself, Given that they will ultimately experience failure, are there some hidden rewards to dieting along the way?" Herman asked. "Sure enough, there are. It turns out that simply declaring you are going on a diet makes you feel better. It seems to bolster people's spirits. They feel that they are empowering themselves. They are already imagining themselves as new and better, taking control of their lives."

Then, when the diet starts, there is the initial thrill of easy victory, that rewarding time when the pounds simply vanish. "You do tend to lose weight. You're fired up," Herman says. Then, of course, the weight loss stalls. And then it reverses.

"When you fail, you have two choices," he continues. "One is to conclude that you didn't try hard enough. Dieters often do that, and the way the diet is structured reinforces that. At the beginning of the diet, when they were pumped up, they lost weight. And later they did not. It is easy to conclude that you must have been easing off. Then, when it is time to start a diet again, it is easy to talk yourself into: 'Well, this time I'm really going to do it. I'm not going to back off.'

"The other choice—and this is the tactic of most diet books—is to say that all your previous diets were based on misconceptions. This diet is based on a new understanding of the principles of metabolism or some other cockamamie thing. What that does is let you say, 'It's true that I failed. But this time it's going to be different.'

"It never is," he added.

I saw all that in the Penn dieters. But what was weird was that

I saw what Herman calls the false hope syndrome in myself as well. I wanted Carmen and Graz, and Jerry and Ron, and all the others to succeed. I wanted it so much that I began to suspend disbelief. I knew, I knew, the science and the overwhelmingly convincing evidence that most obese people will not be able to diet, get thin, and stay at a new low weight. But in those first six months, when everyone was dropping pounds, when Graz lifted her shirt and said to me, "Look, I have a waist!" I fell under the dieters' spell. I allowed myself to think that maybe, just maybe, these people would make it. Maybe they would fulfill their dreams.

I'd often wondered how obesity researchers can keep doing study after study, advertising for subjects like those in the Penn group, starting them off again and again on a path whose outcome they must know for sure. Could it be that the researchers too fall for the dieters' delusion?

What, then, is wrong with this picture? Some scientists, including obesity researchers like Jules Hirsch and Jeff Friedman, suggest an intriguing hypothesis. The origins of people's recent weight gains may have little to do with their current environment or with their willpower, or lack of it, or with today's social customs to snack and eat on the run or with any other popular belief. Instead, they say, we may be a new, heavier human race and our weight may have been set by events that took place very early in life, maybe even prenatally.

Scientists know that animals and people have a range of weights that they can comfortably sustain. Each person's range is different, but any weight much above or below a person's range is almost impossible to maintain. Scientists also know from animal studies that weight as an adult can be affected by early nutrition or infections. They even know that the brain circuits that control eating are modeled and remodeled in mice early in life and again in adolescence.

Maybe, these researchers say, something happened early in life—better nutrition, vaccines to provide freedom from viral infections that plagued children of previous generations, antibiotics to cure infections like strep throat or pneumonia—that precipitated changes in the brain's controls over weight. Maybe a woman who gets sufficient amounts of some vitamin during pregnancy will give birth to a baby with a certain configuration in the brain that leads to a bigger appetite and weight gain.

Higher weights could be an unintended consequence of the nation's generally better health, or maybe even a contributor to it. Maybe whatever is pushing up the average weights of the nation might be for the best. An unfortunate few may end up much, much fatter, massively obese. And others may be unaffected, naturally skinny no matter how hard they try to gain.

It sounds almost surreal. But how real is the notion that soft drinks did this to us (why didn't everyone lose weight when diet sodas came on the market?), or that we're fat because of McDonald's, a chain that has, after all, been around since 1955, when people were much thinner? And does anyone remember those fondue parties of the 1970s, or the way so many of us were enamored of Julia Child's recipes, with their lavish use of butter and cream? And, of course, we used to eat macaroni and cheese and fried fish and Waldorf salads. School lunches then not only provided whole milk and even chocolate milk, but also had squares of frosted cake for dessert. National data say that we now consume less fat and more fruits and vegetables. But, of course, we're fatter.

Or what about the idea that we are more sedentary, in an era that has seen the explosive growth of gyms, surges in the number of people running marathons or going on charity bike rides that can last for hundreds of miles or even walking in shopping malls early in the morning before the stores open? In the 1960s, when people were comparatively thin, one exercise evangelist, Kenneth Cooper, a doctor who coined the word "aerobics," exhorted people to exercise. He said that this was the typical response he heard: "Doc, I don't need much endurance. I work at a desk all day, I watch television at night. I don't exert myself any more than I have to and I have no requirements for exerting myself. Who needs large reserves? Who needs endurance?"

Maybe the lesson is that we've been looking for answers to the obesity epidemic in all the wrong places. At the very least, it does not help to tell people that they are fat, much too fat, and that they just have to eat less and exercise more. After all, as the Penn dieters said at their last meeting, even Oprah gained her weight back, she with all her money and her personal chef and her personal trainer, and with the whole world watching.

I'd like to think also that as the population gets fatter, there might be a rethinking of the risks of a few extra pounds. When health data have not supported the alarmist cries of a medical disaster in the making, could society perhaps let up on the beleaguered fat people?

Then I remember a glossy magazine that was published until the 1990s. It was called *Big Beautiful Woman*, and an anthropologist once gave me a copy, telling me she uses it as a reality check. I flipped through the pages. It was like any other women's magazine except for the models, who were young and attractive but truly fat. At the back of the magazine, I was brought up short. The anthropologist had slipped in a page she had ripped from an ad in a popular fashion magazine. It was a lingerie ad, with a model that was what we have come to expect—extremely slender, much thinner than the average American woman. And the contrast between the model in that ad and the models in the magazine was shocking. Those women in *Big Beautiful Woman* were really fat, I realized, and no amount of pretending that they were fine was going to let them pass in our society. Now, remembering that incident, I recall the diet group meeting when Eva Epstein noted that in some societies, obesity is considered a sign of health. And I remember the man who shot back, "We don't live there."

I also remember Carmen's conclusions about his two years in the diet study, his questioning of whether there ever would be a real solution to his weight problem. I'm not sure there are answers yet for him, except for the ones he's found for himself, to accept that it is hard to be fat in America today and that he will probably be dieting or "monitoring" or trying to diet for the rest of his life.

If nothing else, I believe that research by scientists who have open minds about obesity and its causes and consequences is starting to open doors. I believe that we will see the fruits of that research and that they may not be what we expect or what we hope for. But I also believe that one result will be that the age-old assumption that the perfect diet will somehow emerge will, eventually, fade away.

Notes

PROLOGUE

3 *Three obesity researchers:* Gary D. Foster, interview with the author, Aug. 14, 2003.

3 *"We kept saying, 'Nobody has any data'":* Ibid.

4 *The subjects were randomly assigned:* Robert C. Atkins, *Dr. Atkins' New Diet Revolution* (New York: Avon Books, 2002); also, Kelly Brownell, *The LEARN Program for Weight Management* (Dallas: American Health Publishing Company, 2002).

4 *The Atkins diet, they discovered, seemed better:* Gary D. Foster et al., "A Randomized Trial of a Low-Carbohydrate Diet for Obesity," *New England Journal of Medicine*, May 22, 2003, vol. 348, pp. 2082–2090.

4 *"That's not what we expected," Foster said:* Gary D. Foster, interview with the author, Aug. 14, 2003.

5 *Their paper was accompanied by an editorial:* Robert O. Bonow and Robert H. Eckel, "Diet, Obesity, and Cardiovascular Risk," *New England Journal of Medicine*, May 22, 2003, vol. 348, pp. 2057–2058.

6 *They are like Linda Lee:* Linda Lee, "A Book Made Me Do It: Self-Hypnosis for a Svelter You," *New York Times*, Jan. 4, 2004, sec. 9, p. 9.

6 *The knotty problem was described:* National Academy of Sciences Institute of Medicine, *Weighing the Options: Criteria for Evaluating Weight-Management Programs* (Washington, D.C.: National Academies Press, 1995), p. 37.

6 *He is by no means naturally thin:* Gina Kolata, "No Days Off Are Allowed, Experts Argue," *New York Times*, Oct. 18, 2000, sec. A, p. 1.

1: LOOKING FOR DIETS IN ALL THE WRONG PLACES

9 *If you met Carmen J. Pirollo:* Carmen J. Pirollo's story in this and subsequent chapters is from his statements at the meetings of the diet study and from interviews with the author in 2004, 2005, and 2006.

10 *The three investigators who did:* Gary D. Foster et al., "The Safety and Effectiveness of Low and High Carbohydrate Diets," U.S. National Institutes of Health, http://clinicaltrials.gov/ct/show/NCT00079547.

10 *And it comes with a hefty manual:* Brownell, *The LEARN Program.*

11 *"With Atkins, you'll get the results you've dreamed . . .":* Atkins Nutritionals, Inc., http://www.atkins.com.

11 *"Let's face it—losing weight is hard work . . .":* Brownell, *The LEARN Program,* p. 31.

11 *Atkins says that carbohydrates are diet traps:* Atkins Nutritionals, Inc., http://www.atkins.com.

11 *LEARN says that the source of your calories:* Brownell, *The LEARN Program,* pp. 15–16.

12 *It began about as modestly as a diet can:* Kelly Brownell, interview with the author, Apr. 29, 2004.

13 *Brownell's dissertation went smoothly:* Kelly D. Brownell, "The Effect of Couples Training and Partner Cooperativeness in the Behavioral Treatment of Obesity," *Behaviour Research and Therapy,* vol. 16, pp. 323–333.

13 *"One of the most interesting":* Kelly Brownell, interview with the author, Apr. 29, 2004.

14 *"Diet books have a short half-life":* Ibid.

14 *And scattered little boxes of text give:* Brownell, *The LEARN Program,* p. 16.

15 *In 1973, the American Medical Association's Council on Foods and Nutrition:* "A Critique of Low-Carbohydrate Ketogenic Weight Reduction Regimens: A Review of Dr. Atkins' Diet Revolution," *Journal of the American Medical Association,* June 1973, vol. 224, pp. 1415–1419.

15 *In April 1973, Atkins was called to testify:* Jane E. Brody, "Senate Nutrition Panel to Focus on Perils of Being Overweight," *New York Times,* Apr. 13, 1973, p. 18.

17 *So, in his* New Diet Revolution *he tells of "Tim Wallerdiene":* Robert Atkins, *New Diet Revolution,* p. 9.

17 *Atkins makes exciting promises:* Ibid., p. 1.

17 *"Atkins works because . . .":* Ibid., p. 21.

18 *sales of books promoting low-carbohydrate diets:* Daniel Kadlec, "The Low-Carb Frenzy," *Time,* May 3, 2004, p. 48.

18 *"Obese people get a level of abuse . . .":* Jeffrey Friedman, interview with the author, Apr. 15, 2004.

22 *Weintraub assumed the drugs were safe:* Gina Kolata, "How Phen-Fen, a Diet 'Miracle,' Rose and Fell," *New York Times,* Sept. 23, 1997, sec. F, p. 1.

23 *Finally, in July 1992, the work appeared:* Michael Weintraub, "Long-Term Weight Control," *Clinical Pharmacology & Therapeutics,* May 1992, vol. 51, no. 5, pp. 586–646.

23 *Ben Z. Krentzman, a family practitioner:* Gina Kolata, "Drugs Found to Keep Lost Flab Off," *New York Times,* July 5, 1992, p. 12.

23 *Pietr Hitzig, a doctor in Timonium, Maryland:* Ibid.

23 *Dennis Tison, a Sacramento psychiatrist:* Ibid.

23 *Commercial weight loss centers also gave out the drugs:* Ibid.

23 *"This is L.A.," said Aaron Baumann:* Ibid.

23 *Jenny Craig provided phen-fen to clients, and NutriSystem advertised two months:* Ibid.

23 *The Internet bristled with phen-fen advertisements:* Ibid.

24 *Many doctors, including Hitzig and Krentzman, prescribed them:* Ibid.

24 *Baumann, of California Medical Weight Loss Associates, said:* Gina Kolata, "Diet Pills: Allure and Risk," *New York Times,* July 6, 1977, sec. C, p. 19.

24 *Even university medical centers:* Kolata, "How Phen-Fen," sec. F, p. 1.

24 *In 1996 alone, doctors:* Gina Kolata, "2 Top Diet Drugs Are Recalled Amid Reports of Heart Defects," *New York Times,* Sept. 16, 1997, sec. A, p. 1.

24 *"In truth, I never thought . . .":* Kolata, "How Phen-Fen," sec. F, p. 1.

24 *In July 1997 . . . doctors at the Mayo Clinic:* Kolata, "2 Top Diet Drugs," sec. A, p. 1.

25 *The Food and Drug Administration (FDA) asked doctors:* Ibid.

25 *And Wyeth, while denying that the drugs:* Reed Abelson and Jonathan D. Glater, "A Texas Jury Rules Against a Diet Drug," *New York Times,* Apr. 28, 2004, sec. C, p. 1.

2: EPIPHANIES AND HUCKSTERS

32 *Dieting, of course, is not the image:* Robert Fogel, University of Chicago, interview with the author, Sept. 13, 2005.

32 *Magazines published cruel digs:* K. A. Sanborn, *The Galaxy,* Sept. 1872, vol. 14, no. 3, pp. 426, 429–430.

33 *It was the age of businessman James Buchanan Brady:* "'Diamond Jim' Brady Dies While Asleep," *New York Times,* May 14, 1917, p. 13.

33 *These music hall performers were derided as "beefy":* Lois W. Banner, *American Beauty* (Chicago: University of Chicago Press, 1983), p. 58.

33 *Levenstein relates the story of Oscar Tschirky:* Harvey A. Levenstein, *Revolution at the Table: The Transformation of the American Diet* (New York: Oxford University Press, 1988), p. 13; also, "Food History," http://www.kitchenproject .com, retrieved Sept. 4, 2006, and Cornell University Library, Division of Rare and Manuscript Collections, http://rmc.library.cornell.edu/food/elegant_table/ Oscar_of_the_Waldorf_L.htm.

34 *Fashion decreed that they be thin enough:* Lois W. Banner, *American Beauty,* p. 56.

35 *Byron's constant battle:* Fiona MacCarthy, *Byron: Life and Legend* (New York: Farrar, Straus and Giroux, 2002), p. 62.

35 *Edward John Trelawny, a fierce competitor of Byron's:* Edward J. Trelawny, *Recollections of the Last Days of Shelley and Byron* (London: Henry Frowde, 1906), chap. 6. Available from http://engphil.astate.edu/gallery/Trelawn.html.

Edited and scanned by Jeffrey D. Hoeper, English Dept., Arkansas State University.

35 *Historian Lois Banner notes:* Lois Banner, *American Beauty,* p. 62.

35 *Her name was Louise:* Jean Anthelme Brillat-Savarin, *The Physiology of Taste,* trans. by M.F.K. Fisher (New York: Counterpoint Press, 1971), pp. 253–255.

36 *He himself had a weight problem:* Ibid., p. 237.

36 *While some are more prone to obesity:* Ibid., p. 245.

36 *A "Fat Lady," for example:* Ibid., p. 239.

36 *Observations like that, he said:* Ibid., pp. 250–251.

37 *"It has rightly been said":* Ibid., p. 241.

37 *He knew what sort of response that would get:* Ibid., p. 251.

37 *"M. Louis Greffulhe, who was later honored . . .":* Ibid., pp. 248–249.

38 *Banting told his story in a surprise international bestseller:* William Banting, *Letter on Corpulence Addressed to the Public,* 4th ed. (London: Pall Mall bookseller to the Queen, 1865), pp. 1–19. Available from Atkins Diet & Low Carbohydrate Support, http://www.lowcarb.ca/corpulence.

40 *He gave away the first two thousand copies of his pamphlet:* Ibid., preface.

40 *The pamphlet went through twelve editions:* Lois W. Banner, *American Beauty,* p. 129.

40 *Others criticized Harvey's complicity:* "Banting on Corpulence," *Blackwood's Magazine,* reprinted in *The Living Age,* Dec. 10, 1864, vol. 1071, pp. 555, 559, 561.

41 *When the fourth edition of Banting's book was published:* Banting, *Letter on Corpulence,* introduction.

41 *Decades later, in 1895,* The New York Times *needed: New York Times,* June 21, 1895, p. 4.

41 *Some tried ipecac:* Hillel Schwartz, *Never Satisfied: A Cultural History of Diets, Fantasies, and Fat* (New York: Free Press, 1986), pp. 97–98.

42 *Brillat-Savarin said the problem with exercise:* Brillat-Savarin, *Physiology of Taste,* p. 250.

42 *In the nineteenth century, the health food diet:* James C. Whorton, *Crusaders for Fitness: The History of American Health Reformers* (Princeton, N.J.: Princeton University Press, 1982), p. 38.

42 *His disciples became obsessed with their weight:* Schwartz, *Never Satisfied,* pp. 26–27.

42 *He insisted that people could rise above hunger:* Ibid., p. 31.

42 *Graham told his followers that they should eat simple foods:* Schwartz, *Never Satisfied,* pp. 25–26, 44–45; also, Whorton, *Crusaders for Fitness,* p. 47.

42 *Graham's close associate, the Boston health reformer William A. Alcott:* Schwartz, *Never Satisfied,* p. 44.

43 *They wrote letters and testimonials:* Ibid., p. 27.

43 *Dinner at a Graham house must feature such delicacies:* Whorton, *Crusaders for Fitness,* p. 59.

43 *One satirist of the time:* Schwartz, *Never Satisfied,* p. 27.

43 *In 1840, students and faculty at Oberlin College:* Whorton, *Crusaders for Fitness*, pp. 126–127.

43 *and the townspeople became distressed by stories:* Schwartz, *Never Satisfied*, p. 45.

44 *The year was 1889:* Whorton, *Crusaders for Fitness*, p. 170.

44 *As Sylvester Graham's associate William A. Alcott wrote:* Whorton, *Crusaders for Fitness*, p. 174.

44 *A British visitor wrote:* Schwartz, *Never Satisfied*, p. 42.

44 *Even women were virtually inhaling:* Ibid., p. 42.

44 *As proof of his method:* Whorton, *Crusaders for Fitness*, p. 178.

45 *"With no special training in the interim . . .":* Ibid., p. 183.

45 *Fletcher became known as "The Great Masticator":* Schwartz, *Never Satisfied*, p. 125.

45 *"In obtaining Fletcherism, I found myself aided greatly . . .":* Goodwin Brown, "What Is Right and Wrong in the Use of Food," *New York Times Sunday Magazine*, June 23, 1907, p. 5.

45 *Fletcher gained celebrity endorsements:* Schwartz, *Never Satisfied*, p. 126.

46 *Cookbook author and magazine columnist Sarah Tyson Rorer:* Ibid., p. 126.

46 *Henry James, the American expatriate writer:* Schwartz, *Never Satisfied*, pp. 126, 134; also, Whorton, *Crusaders for Fitness*, p. 198.

46 *"Fletcher seemed willing to devote . . .":* Levenstein, *Revolution at the Table*, p. 88.

47 *The scientists put forth a bold-faced plea:* Ibid.

47 *But, asked Chittenden, who directed:* Whorton, *Crusaders for Fitness*, p. 184.

47 *In Fletcher, Chittenden found what seemed like the perfect subject:* Schwartz, *Never Satisfied*, p. 131.

47 *That seemingly meager portion was anathema:* Whorton, *Crusaders for Fitness*, p. 188.

47 *(Today, the National Academy of Sciences . . .):* Available from Institute of Medicine, http://www.iom.edu/Object.File/Master/21/372/0.pdf.

48 *Fletcher moved in with Chittenden:* Whorton, *Crusaders for Fitness*, p. 185.

48 *"To me the chewing business became unimportant . . .":* Ibid., p. 187.

48 *When Yale's physical education expert, William G. Anderson:* Ibid., p. 185.

48 *But Chittenden, who kept careful track of what Fletcher ate:* "Mr. Fletcher Again Explained," *New York Times*, Jan. 7, 1908, p. 6.

48 *Doctors warned him that it was risky:* Levenson, *Revolution at the Table*, pp. 90–91.

49 *He decided to expand the study:* Ibid.

49 *For sedentary people, or "brain workers," as he called them:* Ibid.

49 *The army was interested because:* Ibid.

49 *From the fall of 1903 until the summer of 1904:* Whorton, *Crusaders for Fitness*, p. 189.

49 *But in Chittenden's studies, no one's health declined:* Ibid.

49 *"In presenting the results of the experiments, herein described . . ."*: Available from Sportscience: A Peer Reviewed Site for Sports Research, http://www.sportsci.org/news/history/chittenden/chittenden.html#chit1.

50 *"In general, it may be said that whatever the explanation . . ."*: "Vegetarians the Stronger: Yale's Flesh-Eating Athletes Beaten in Severe Endurance Tests," *New York Times*, Mar. 22, 1907, p. 3.

50 *Instead, he said, the experiments*: "Eat for Strength," Seventh Day Adventist Reform Movement, Northwest U.S. Field, available from http://www.sdarm.net/northwestfield/eatbody.htm.

50 The New York Times *reviewed the book*: "What New Yorkers Eat vs. What They Should," *New York Times*, June 2, 1907, p. SM3.

51 *In 1907, he informed a convention of home economists*: Levenstein, *Revolution at the Table*, p. 91.

51 *In 1908,* The Medical Record *published an article*: "Mr. Fletcher Again Explained," p. 6.

51 *By the time Fletcher died, in 1919, of a heart attack*: Levenstein, *Revolution at the Table*, p. 95.

52 *The mistake many make is to think*: Irving Fisher and Eugene Lyman Fisk, *How to Live: Rules for Healthful Living Based on Modern Science* (New York: Funk and Wagnalls, 1916), p. 33.

52 *telling themselves that "many articles . . ."*: Ibid., p. 33.

52 *"Constant vigilance is necessary . . ."*: Ibid., p. 34.

52 *In the end, they say, "the reduction of weight . . ."*: Ibid., p. 218.

52 *"Why do physicians take so much care . . . ?"*: "To Make Outdoor Sleeping Easy and Popular," *New York Times*, May 26, 1907, p. SM4.

52 *Mail-order hucksters were preying on*: "Anti-Fat Cures Branded as 'Fakes,'" *New York Times*, Aug. 5, 1914, p. 15.

53 *Soon calorie-counting was the new, preferred method*: Schwartz, *Never Satisfied*, p. 140.

53 *In 1918, the bestseller* Diet and Health, with Key to the Calories, *appeared*: Ibid., pp. 175–176.

54 *And, notes Levenstein, "The Dessert hotel chain of the Pacific Northwest . . ."*: Levenstein, *Revolution at the Table*, p. 191.

54 *A cookbook of the era,* Food and How to Cook It, *noted*: Ibid., p. 166.

54 *Even young teenagers, who used to be less affected*: Joan Jacobs Brumberg, *The Body Project: An Intimate History of American Girls* (New York: Random House, 1977), p. 99.

54 *She tells of a Chicago teenager, Yvonne Blue*: Ibid., p. 100.

55 *She sent away for a diet book*: Ibid., pp. 104–106.

55 *She kept the weight off and proudly reported*: Ibid.

55 *The contest took place in New York City in 1921*: "Pills Make a Fat Contestant Fatter," *New York Times*, Oct. 27, 1921, p. 14.

55 *He advised women what to eat*: "Fair Fat Reducers Balk at Taking Oil," *New York Times*, Oct. 28, 1921, p. 16.

56 *The dieters sang Copeland's praises at first:* "In Training Five Days Can Lace Her Shoes," *New York Times,* Oct. 22, 1921, p. 6.

56 *Four months later,* The New York Times *reported:* "Fat Women Hold Graduates' Reunion," *New York Times,* Jan. 18, 1922, p. 16.

56 *A decade later, he was fat again:* "Hoover Is Thinner and in Glowing Health," *New York Times,* Jan. 29, 1932, p. 1.

56 *Even that austere prescription was not enough:* Schwartz, *Never Satisfied,* p. 177.

57 *That was the advice in a bestselling book:* Robert Linn, *The Last Chance Diet—When Everything Else Has Failed, Dr. Linn's Protein-Sparing Fast Program* (New York: Lyle Stuart, 1977).

57 *"It is much easier to sit at a dinner party . . .":* Judith Weintraub, "An Empty Plate on Every Table," *New York Times,* May 18, 1977, p. 58.

57 *All along there were the strange diets:* Schwartz, *Never Satisfied,* p. 198–199.

57 *Special diet drinks also came and went:* Ibid.

57 *the "fabulous formula,"* Ladies' Home Journal *called it:* Ibid., p. 198.

58 *"We keep coming back to the same kinds of diets . . .":* Hillel Schwartz, interview with the author, Feb. 19, 2004.

58 *Even obesity surgery dates back to the early twentieth century:* "Under Knife for Obesity," *New York Times,* Nov. 11, 1911, p. 1.

58 *In 1922, Dr. Max Thorek of Chicago:* Schwartz, *Never Satisfied,* p. 178; also, "Dr. Max Thorek, Physician, Was 79," *New York Times,* Jan. 27, 1960, p. 33.

58 *The first of these diet clubs was TOPS:* "Take Off Pounds Sensibly," available from http://www.tops.org/ReadArticle.asp?articleId=1203.

58 *Others followed—such as Overeaters Anonymous in 1960:* Overeaters Anonymous, http://www.oa.org/about_oa.html.

59 *The next year, Weight Watchers was founded:* Weight Watchers, http://www.weightwatchers.com/about/his/history.aspx.

59 *Jenny Craig, founded in Australia in 1983:* Jenny Craig, http://www.jennycraig.com/corporate/news/fact_sheet.asp.

59 *People tried everything:* Schwartz, *Never Satisfied,* pp. 196–197. About ephedra's removal from the market in 2004, see Food and Drug Administration, http://www.fda.gov/oc/initiatives/ephedra/december2003/advisory.html.

3: OH, TO BE AS THIN AS JENNIFER ANISTON (OR BRAD PITT)

65 *When asked, "Would you like to weigh less?":* Katherine Flegal, personal communication, February 9, 2006; unpublished data from the Centers for Disease Control and Prevention's National Health and Nutrition Examination Survey III.

65 *Jennifer Aniston, for example, reportedly is:* Allstarz.org, http://www.allstarz.org/aniston/profile.html.

65 *And it makes her officially underweight:* Centers for Disease Control and Prevention, http://www.cdc.gov/nchs/data/ad/ad330.pdf.

65 *"The perfect Miss America is supposedly 5'8" and 110 pounds":* iVillage.com, http://beauty.ivillage.com/0,,ms09-1,00.html.

66 *But when one nutritionist, Benjamin Caballero:* Sharon Rubinstein, "Is Miss America an Undernourished Role Model?" *Journal of the American Medical Association,* Mar. 2000, vol. 283, p. 1569.

67 *He reportedly is 6 feet tall and weighs 159 pounds:* Allstarz.org, http://www .bradpittfan.com/bio.htm.

67 *Studies have found that fat people are less likely to be admitted to elite colleges:* Yale University Rudd Center, http://www.yaleruddcenter.org; also, Gina Kolata, "The Burdens of Being Overweight: Mistreatment and Misconceptions," *New York Times,* Nov. 22, 1992, p. A1.

68 *According to Yale University's Rudd Center:* Yale University Rudd Center, http://www.yaleruddcenter.org.

68 *Tina Hedberg of Conover, Wisconsin:* Tina Hedberg, telephone interview with the author, Sept. 19, 2005.

68 *Miriam Berg, president of the Council on Size and Weight Discrimination:* Miriam Berg, telephone interview with the author, Sept. 19, 2005.

69 *In one now-classic study, Colleen Rand:* Kolata, "The Burdens of Being Overweight," p. A1.

69 *Esther Rothblum, a professor of women's studies:* Ibid.

70 *"Overweight people have a condition . . .":* Ibid.

70 *"There's that implicit assumption . . .":* Ibid.

70 *She was larger than life:* Carolyn Kitch, *The Girl on the Magazine Cover: The Origins of Visual Stereotypes in American Mass Media* (Chapel Hill, N.C.: University of North Carolina Press, 2001), pp. 37–44; also, Banner, *American Beauty,* p. 155.

70 *There she is again, sitting on a grassy bank:* Banner, *American Beauty,* fig. 22.

71 *"We perceive that there is something to conquer . . .":* Kitch, *The Girl on the Magazine Cover,* p. 44.

71 *"Her clothes, her hats, her walk and her indescribable chic . . .":* Henry Collins Brown, "In the Golden Nineties" (Hastings on Hudson, N.Y.: Valentine's Manual, 1928, c. 1927), p. 186. Available from http://www.hti.umich .edu/m/moa/.

71 *Before her arrival, wrote a reporter for the* New York World: Kitch, *The Girl on the Magazine Cover,* p. 37.

71 *In 1909, they would parade down New York's Fifth Avenue:* Marc Debrol, "'Jeunes Américaines': A French Writer Tells How American Girls Appear to Frenchmen and Why This Country's 'Daughters of the Rich' Are Typical of the Race," *New York Times Sunday Magazine,* Oct. 17, 1909, p. SM5.

71 *"The Gibson Girl is to be found in homes . . .":* Banner, *American Beauty,* p. 154.

71 *"The Gibson Girl, we trust, is but a passing fancy . . .":* "Gibson Girl vs. English Girl," *New York Times,* Nov. 19, 1908, p. 8.

71 *By 1907, reporters were noting:* "American Beauty Under Discussion," *New York Times,* Sept. 22, 1907, p. C1.

72 *"From hundreds, thousands, tens of thousands, I formed my idea . . .":* Edward Marshall, "The Gibson Girl Analyzed by Her Originator," *New York Times*, Nov. 20, 1910, p. SM6.

72 *In 1903, Collier's magazine paid Gibson $100,000:* Kitch, *The Girl on the Magazine Cover*, p. 39. Information on currency values available at http://www.bls.gov/.

72 *Gibson insisted that the phenomenon had taken him by surprise:* William Griffith, "The Gibson Girl's Creator and American Girl Types," *New York Times*, Apr. 30, 1905, p. SM4.

72 *Even actresses like Lillian Russell, one of the great beauties:* Banner, *American Beauty*, p. 151.

73 *"Any girl that looks back and sees . . .":* Maude Radford Warren, "American Beauty Handmade in America," *New York Times*, Mar. 26, 1921, p. 46.

73 *In 1912, reports historian Lois Banner, the daughter of an actress:* Banner, *American Beauty*, p. 153.

73 *Within a few years of creating the Gibson Girl:* Kitch, *The Girl on the Magazine Cover*, p. 40.

73 *young men who showed up in society columns:* Lois Banner, *American Beauty*, pp. 243–245.

73 *They had their own clubs:* "The Ball of the Heavyweights: A Jovial Gathering at Irving Hall," *New York Times*, Jan. 24, 1875, p. 5; also, "Fat Men and Clams," *New York Times*, Aug. 15, 1879, p. 8.

73 *Now the clubs were shuttered:* Schwartz, *Never Satisfied*, p. 88.

73 *They gossiped about how:* Ibid., p. 90.

74 *One day, Chauncey Depew, a senator from New York:* Ibid.

74 *At first he succeeded and proudly wore:* Ibid., pp. 90, 111.

74 *Now they wanted to look:* Kitch, *The Girl on the Magazine Cover*, p. 122.

74 *Kitch describes the flapper in Held's drawings:* Ibid., pp. 121–122.

74 *(Kitch also explains the origin of the word . . .):* Ibid., p. 132.

75 *They made scales that were pretty much the same:* Ibid., pp. 163–165.

76 *"The 19th-century advertisements for platform scales . . .":* Ibid., p. 170.

76 *In the nineteenth century, mirrors, known as "looking glasses":* Joan Jacobs Brumberg, Cornell University, telephone interview with the author, 2003.

77 *For the first time, the technology of photography:* Jan Todd, University of Texas at Austin, telephone interview with the author, 2003.

77 *"An excess of flesh is to be looked upon . . .":* Schwartz, *Never Satisfied*, p. 96.

77 *The winner of a 1904 contest in New York:* Gina Kolata, *Ultimate Fitness: The Quest for Truth About Exercise and Health* (New York: Farrar, Straus and Giroux, 2003), pp. 38–39.

77 *Historian Lois Banner remarks, "It must be made clear . . .":* Banner, *American Beauty*, p. 153.

78 *Even Marilyn Monroe, the archetypical voluptuous woman:* Marilyn Monroe .com, http://www.marilynmonroe.com/about/facts.html.

78	*"By the 1960s," writes historian Carolyn Kitch:* Kitch, *The Girl on the Magazine Cover*, p. 185.

78	*She was 5 feet 7 inches tall and reportedly weighed 91 pounds:* http://www .shapesforwomen.com/articles/history.asp, accessed October 30, 2006.

4: A VOICE IN THE WILDERNESS

86	*His long odyssey began in the late 1940s:* Albert J. Stunkard's ideas are taken from telephone interviews with and e-mails to the author in 2004 and 2005 and from Stunkard's published papers.

86	*One day, Maxine timidly crept in:* Albert J. Stunkard, "Eating Disorders and Obesity," in *Progress in Obesity Research*, 1999, vol. 8, B. Guy-Grand and G. Ailhaud, editors (John Libbey & Co: 8th International Congress on Obesity, 1999), p. 243.

86	*"Little advice was forthcoming . . .":* Ibid., p. 244.

87	*Then, shortly afterward, another fat patient:* Ibid., p. 245.

88	*"he drove through heavy midtown New York traffic . . .":* Ibid.

90	*One popular notion, advanced in the 1950s:* Hilda Bruch with Grace Tourraine, "Obesity in Childhood: V. The Family Frame of Obese Children," *Psychosomatic Medicine*, Jan./Feb. 1940, vol. 2, no. 1, pp. 141–206.

90	*"There were all sorts of ideas as to how . . .":* Albert J. Stunkard, "Beginners Mind: Trying to Learn Something about Obesity," *Annals of Behavioral Medicine*, 1991, vol. 13, pp. 22, 52.

90	*He began with a small pilot study:* Ibid.; also, N. Weinberg, M. Mendelson, and A. J. Stunkard, "A Failure to Find Distinctive Personality Features in a Group of Obese Men," *American Journal of Psychiatry*, 1961, vol. 117, pp. 1035–1037.

92	*Obese people were slightly more neurotic:* Stunkard, "Beginners Mind," p. 53.

92	*The incidence of obesity was 30 percent:* P. B. Goldblatt, M. E. Moore, A. J. Stunkard, "Social Factors in Obesity," *Journal of the American Medical Association*, 1965, vol. 192, pp. 1039–1044.

94	*"I began to ask my obese patients about how they ate":* Stunkard, "Beginners Mind," p. 52.

95	*He estimates that the condition occurs in just 1.5 percent:* Albert J. Stunkard and Kelly Costello Allison, "Two Forms of Disordered Eating in Obesity: Binge Eating and Night Eating," *International Journal of Obesity*, 2003, vol. 27, pp. 1–12.

96	*Its proponents say it afflicts about 2 percent:* Albert J. Stunkard and Kelly C. Allison, "Binge Eating Disorder: Disorder or Marker?" *International Journal of Eating Disorders*, 2003, vol. 34, p. S108.

96	*It is listed in the psychiatry manual as a "provisional diagnosis":* Erica Goode, "Watching Volunteers, Experts Seek Clues to Eating Disorders," *New York Times*, Oct. 24, 2000, p. F1.

96	*but when Stunkard and others did rigorous studies:* Stunkard and Allison, "Binge Eating Disorder," p. S113.

96 *"If you actually talk with people who have binge eating disorder . . .":* Goode, "Watching Volunteers," p. F1.

96 *"Outside North America, it's basically a laugh":* Ibid.

98 *The LEARN manual has a section:* Brownell, *The LEARN Program,* pp. 25–27.

99 *"Many overweight people have trouble . . .":* Ibid., pp. 26–27.

99 *That's also the message when the manual asks:* Ibid., p. 37.

5: A DRIVE TO EAT

107 *During World War II a remarkable experiment began:* Ancel Keys et al., *The Biology of Human Starvation,* 2 vols. (Minneapolis: University of Minnesota Press, 1950).

108 *Keys wrote: "Those who ate in the common dining room . . .":* Ibid., p. 833.

108 *The men "often reported that they got . . .":* Ibid., p. 834.

108 *They struggled over urges: to "gulp their food down ravenously":* Ibid., p. 835.

108 *Some of the men began collecting cooking implements:* Ibid., p. 837.

108 *"Several men were unable to adhere to their diets . . .":* Ibid., p. 884.

109 *Keys went on: "While working in a grocery store . . .":* Ibid., p. 887.

109 *One man wrote, "I am one of about three or four . . .":* Ibid., p. 853.

109 *One man's meals had as many as 5,000 to 6,000 calories:* Ibid., p. 843.

109 *Keys describes the scene:* Ibid., p. 847.

110 *One prisoner, Private First Class Risto Milosevich:* Alex Kershaw, *The Longest Winter: The Battle of the Bulge and the Epic Story of WWII's Most Decorated Platoon* (New York: Da Capo Press, 2004), p. 188.

110 *The Rockefeller scientist was Jules Hirsch:* Jules Hirsch's research and views on obesity are based on interviews with and e-mails to the author in 2004 and 2005 and on his published papers.

113 *One man, C.F., was thirty-eight and weighed 350 pounds:* Myron L. Glucksman and Jules Hirsch, "The Response of Obese Patients to Weight Reduction: A Clinical Evaluation of Behavior," *Psychosomatic Medicine,* 1968, vol. 30, no. 1, pp. 1–11.

115 *The Rockefeller subjects also had a psychiatric syndrome:* Myron L. Glucksman et al., "The Response of Obese Patients to Weight Reduction: II. A Quantitative Evaluation of Behavior," *Psychosomatic Medicine,* 1968, vol. 30, no. 4, pp. 359–373.

115 *"Perhaps the most intriguing aspect of this study . . .":* Ibid., p. 317.

115 *Eventually, more than fifty people:* Jules Hirsch, "Obesity: Matter over Mind?" *Cerebrum: The Dana Forum on Brain Science,* Winter 2003, vol. 5, no. 1, p. 16.

116 *Sims says he got the idea from research he had done:* Ethan Sims's research and views on obesity are from his publications and interviews with the author in 2004.

119 *In a review article published in 1976, Sims wrote:* Ethan A. H. Sims, "Experimental Obesity, Dietary-Induced Thermogenesis, and Their Clinical Implications," *Clinics in Endocrinology and Metabolism,* July 1976, vol. 5, no. 2, p. 386.

119 *Hirsch wrote his own summary of the work:* Hirsch, "Obesity: Matter Over Mind?" p. 15.

122 *The results, published in 1986, were unequivocal:* Albert J. Stunkard et al., "An Adoption Study of Human Obesity," *New England Journal of Medicine,* Jan. 23, 1986, vol. 314, pp. 193–198.

122 *The scientists summarized their data:* Ibid., p. 195; also, T.I.A. Sorensen, C. Holst, and A. J. Stunkard, "Childhood Body Mass Index—Genetic and Familial Environmental Influences Assessed in a Longitudinal Adoption Study," *International Journal of Obesity,* 1992, vol. 16, pp. 705–714.

122 *"Current efforts to prevent obesity . . .":* Stunkard et al., "An Adoption Study of Human Obesity," p. 197.

122 *A few years later, Stunkard conducted another study:* Albert J. Stunkard et al., "The Body-Mass Index of Twins Who Have Been Reared Apart," *New England Journal of Medicine,* May 24, 1990, vol. 322, no. 21, pp. 1483–1487.

123 *"almost all of the differences . . .":* Gina Kolata, "Where Fat Is the Problem, Heredity Is the Answer, Studies Find," *New York Times,* May 24, 1990, p. B9.

124 *"We definitely have some very efficient people . . .":* Ibid.

124 *Stunkard said the two studies together gave a scientific reason:* Ibid.

125 *Jeffrey Friedman, an obesity researcher at Rockefeller:* J. M. Friedman, "A War on Obesity, Not the Obese," *Science,* Feb. 7, 2003, vol. 299, no. 5608, pp. 856–858.

6: INSATIABLE, VORACIOUS APPETITES

132 *The child was born in 1887 and was slim until March 1899:* Hilda Bruch, "The Froehlich Syndrome: Report of the Original Case," *American Journal of Diseases of Children,* 1939, vol. 58, pp. 1282, 1283, 1285.

132 *"In the depth of the sphenoid sinus . . .":* Ibid., p. 1282.

133 *He insisted that the condition was extremely rare:* Schwartz, *Never Satisfied,* pp. 290–291.

133 *The first paper appeared in the* Anatomical Record: A. W. Hetherington and S. W. Ranson, "Hypothalamic Lesions and Adiposity in the Rat," *Anatomical Record,* Oct. 1940, vol. 78, p. 149–172.

133 *"The pair of lesions on either side . . .":* Ibid., p. 151.

133 *Their autopsies revealed that the rats:* Ibid., p. 157.

134 *The rats, the scientists reported, "voraciously gnawed . . .":* John R. Brombeck, Jay Tepperman, and C.N.H. Long, "Experimental Hypothalamic Hyperphagia in the Albino Rat," *Yale Journal of Biology and Medicine,* 1943, vol. 15, p. 835.

134 *When they autopsied the rat that died:* Ibid., p. 835.

134 *It was an effect so striking that it became almost legendary:* Robert Pool, *Fat: Fighting the Obesity Epidemic* (Oxford: Oxford University Press, 2001), p. 51.

134 *The rats were eating three times as much as normal animals:* Brombeck et al., "Experimental Hypothalamic Hyperphagia," p. 835.

134 *The animals were not picky eaters:* Ibid., p. 848.

134 *"Many of the animals were almost incredibly obese . . .":* Ibid., p. 845.

134 *Their livers were so full of fat:* Ibid., p. 846.

135 *The earliest published report:* Pool, *Fat,* p. 49.

135 *Steven B. Heymsfield, who was the deputy director of the Obesity Research Center:* Gina Kolata, "The Fat Epidemic: How the Body Knows When to Gain or Lose," *New York Times,* Oct. 17, 2000, p. F1.

136 *It was found by a caretaker at the Jackson Laboratory:* Ellen Ruppel Shell, *The Hungry Gene: The Inside Story of the Obesity Industry* (New York: Grove Press, 2002), p. 57.

136 *A graduate student came to take a look:* Ibid.

136 *Then, sixteen years later, in 1965, another strain of mutant mice:* Pool, *Fat,* p. 96.

136 *The strain of mice, named* db *(pronounced "dee-bee"), for "diabetes":* Katherine P. Hummel, Margaret M. Dickie, and Douglas L. Coleman, "Diabetes, a New Mutation in the Mouse," *Science,* Sept. 2, 1966, vol. 153, pp. 1127–1128.

136 *The operation involved slicing one animal open:* Pool, *Fat,* pp. 104–105.

137 *So he blamed himself when his first few conjoined mouse pairs died:* Pool, *Fat,* p. 106; also, Schell, *The Hungry Gene,* p. 60.

137 *But those normal mice were no longer normal:* Pool, *Fat,* p. 106.

137 *Coleman had no idea what was happening:* Pool, *Fat,* p. 106; also, Schell, *The Hungry Gene,* p. 61.

139 *Coleman published his work in 1973:* D. L. Coleman and K. P. Hummel, "The Influence of Genetic Background on the Expression of the Obese (*ob*) Gene in the Mouse," *Diabetologia,* 1973, vol. 9, pp. 287–293.

140 *"At the time, a lot of people didn't think ob mice . . .":* Jeffrey Friedman of Rockefeller University, interview with the author, Apr. 20, 2004.

140 *Back when he was just starting out in science:* Jeffrey Friedman's story is from interviews with the author in 2004 and 2005.

141 *one of Friedman's colleagues:* Bruce Schneider, interview with the author, May 18, 2004.

142 *Rozin likes to devise little experiments:* Paul Rozin, interviews with and e-mails to the author in 2004 and 2005.

143 *In one experiment, Wansink asked:* Brian Wansink, *Mindless Eating: Why We Eat More Than We Think* (New York: Bantam Books, 2006), pp. 16–19.

145 *"I weighed myself every day . . .":* Bruce Schneider, interview with the author, May 18, 2004.

7: THE GIRL WHO HAD NO LEPTIN

157 *She was born in 1989 to Pakistani parents:* I. S. Farooqi et al., "Brief Report: Effects of Recombinant Leptin Therapy in a Child with Congenital Leptin Deficiency," *New England Journal of Medicine,* Sept. 16, 1999, vol. 341, pp. 879–884; also, Stephen O'Rahilly, interview with the author, Apr. 13, 2005.

159 *No one, he says, can consciously calibrate food intake:* Jeffrey Friedman's thoughts on leptin are from interviews with the author in 2004 and 2005.

160 *The answer was that the leptin gene in ob mice:* Yiying Zhang et al., "Positional Cloning of the Mouse *Obese* Gene and Its Human Homologue," *Nature*, Dec. 1, 1994, vol. 372, pp. 425–432.

161 *They published the results in the journal* Science *in July 1995:* Jeffrey L. Halaas et al., "Weight-Reducing Effects of the Plasma Protein Encoded by the *Obese* Gene," *Science*, July 28, 1995, vol. 269, pp. 543–546.

161 *"When you are talking about 0.67 percent . . .":* Gina Kolata, "Fat Signaling Hormone Is Clue to Weight Control," *New York Times*, Aug. 1, 1995, p. C1.

161 *In a paper published alongside Friedman's:* L. A. Campfield et al., "Recombinant Mouse OB Protein: Evidence for a Peripheral Signal Linking Adiposity and Central Neural Networks," *Science*, July 28, 1995, vol. 269, pp. 546–549.

161 *Philip Gordon, who was then the director:* Gina Kolata, "Researchers Find Hormone Causes a Loss of Weight," *New York Times*, July 27, 1995, p. A1.

162 *The leptin discovery, said Theodore Van Itallie:* Ibid.

162 *Mickey Stunkard called the results "fabulous":* Ibid.

162 *So Rockefeller University, which owned the rights:* Jeffrey Friedman, e-mail to the author, May 30, 2006; also, Gina Kolata, "How the Body Knows When to Gain and Lose," *New York Times*, Oct. 17, 2000, p. F1.

162 *Two and a half years later, in October 1999:* Steven B. Heymsfield et al., "Recombinant Leptin for Weight Loss in Obese and Lean Adults," *Journal of the American Medical Association*, 1999, vol. 282, pp. 1568–1575.

163 *"You would have to look at it and say . . .":* Gina Kolata, "Hormone That Slimmed Fat Mice Disappoints as Panacea in People," *New York Times*, Oct. 27, 1999, p. A1.

163 *"The great hope for leptin has not held up":* Ibid.

163 *Jeff Friedman saw some hope:* E-mail to the author, May 30, 2006.

164 *"Most look at the discovery of leptin . . .":* Steven B. Heymsfield, interviews with the author, Oct. 1999.

164 *The diagrams typically used different colors:* Michael K. Badman and Jeffrey S. Flier, "The Gut and Energy Balance: Visceral Allies in the Obesity Wars," *Science*, Mar. 25, 2005, vol. 307, pp. 1909–1914.

166 *At the University of Pittsburgh:* Author's personal observations, July 3, 2004.

168 *"A lot of thin people . . .":* Stephen O'Rahilly, interview with the author, Feb. 27, 2005.

168 *The discovery of leptin's effects early in life:* Richard Simerly, interview with the author, Mar. 28, 2004.

169 *"Bingo," Simerly said. "The lights went on":* Gina Kolata, "Studies on a Mouse Hormone Bear on Fatness in Humans," *New York Times*, Apr. 2, 2004, p. A14.

169 *Then Friedman and his colleagues discovered that leptin surges:* Ibid.; also, Jeffrey Friedman, interview with the author, Mar. 28, 2004.

169 *The researchers then tested another hormone:* Ibid.

169 *"I'd always imagined this system had a fixed architecture . . .":* Ibid.

170 *"It all comes back to the same issues . . .":* Kolata, "Studies on a Mouse Hormone," p. A14.

171 *Dr. Gregory S. Barsh, of Stanford University:* Kolata, "How the Body Knows," p. F1.

171 *"We think it helps control the long-term . . .":* Ibid.

171 *Or so reasoned Dr. Stephen R. Bloom:* Stephen R. Bloom, interviews with the author, Sept. 2003 and May 6, 2005; also, Gina Kolata, "Study Finds Appetites Reduced by Hormone," *New York Times*, Sept. 4, 2003, p. A16, and Rachel L. Batterham et al., "Inhibition of Food Intake in Obese Subjects by Peptide YY_{3-36}," *New England Journal of Medicine*, Sept. 4, 2003, vol. 349, pp. 941–948.

172 *The rat studies were a bit tricky, Bloom reports:* Stephen R. Bloom, interview with the author, May 6, 2005.

172 *"Medically, it's a disaster to be obese":* Ibid.

172 *But hoary methods like filling up with water:* Batterham et al., "Inhibition of Food Intake," pp. 941–948; also, Stephen R. Bloom, interviews with the author, Sept. 2003 and May 6, 2005.

173 *"Most of us are the same weight year after year":* Stephen R. Bloom, interview with the author, May 6, 2005.

173 *The PYY study was preliminary, but so promising:* Batterham et al., "Inhibition of Food Intake," pp. 941–948.

173 *He started a small company, Thiakis:* Stephen R. Bloom, interview with the author, May 6, 2005.

174 *In the meantime, Bloom switched his attention:* Ibid.

174 *Bloom tried it out with rats:* Ibid.

175 *In the meantime, Bloom did the same sort of study:* Ibid.

175 *O'Rahilly and his colleagues discovered the woman's problem:* R. S. Jackson et al., "Obesity and Impaired Prohormone Processing Associated with Mutations in the Human Prohormone Convertase 1 PC1 Gene," *Nature Genetics*, 1997, vol. 16, pp. 303–306.

176 *She began receiving leptin shots:* I. S. Farooqi et al., "Brief Report: Effects of Recombinant Leptin Therapy in a Child with Congenital Leptin Deficiency," *New England Journal of Medicine*, Sept. 16, 1999, vol. 341, pp. 879–884; also, Stephen O'Rahilly, interview with the author, Apr. 13, 2005.

176 *After a week of leptin injections:* Ibid.

176 *"It was incredibly dramatic," O'Rahilly said:* Kolata, "Hormone That Slimmed Fat Mice," p. A1.

177 *Since then, O'Rahilly and Farooqi have treated four other children:* Stephen O'Rahilly, interview with the author, Apr. 13, 2005.

177 *In one study, Dr. Julio Licinio of the University of California:* Julio Licinio et al., "Phenotypic Effects of Leptin Replacement on Morbid Obesity, Diabetes

Mellitus, Hypogonadism, and Behavior in Leptin-Deficient Adults," *Proceedings of the National Academy of Sciences*, Mar. 30, 2004, vol. 101, no. 13, pp. 4531–4536.

177 *O'Rahilly and Farooqi, though, who have treated:* Stephen O'Rahilly, interview with the author, May 31, 2006.

178 *They put out a call to doctors worldwide:* Stephen O'Rahilly, interview with the author, Apr. 13, 2005.

178 *"You really can't ignore that data":* Ibid.

178 *But despite the studies dating back twenty years:* Ibid.

179 *The most common so far is melanocortin-4 receptor deficiency:* I. S. Farooqi et al., "Clinical Spectrum of Obesity and Mutations in the Melanocortin-4 Receptor Gene," *New England Journal of Medicine*, Mar. 20, 2003, vol. 348, pp. 1085–1095.

179 *The children are tall and very fat:* Ibid.

179 *Not only did O'Rahilly and Farooqi find children:* Ibid.

180 *"People don't like the genetics of behavior":* Stephen O'Rahilly, interview with the author, Apr. 13, 2005.

180 *"I'm a big guy, and I'll never forget . . .":* Ibid.

180 *"It is really bad to be morbidly obese":* Ibid.

8: THE FAT WARS

188 *He told* The New York Times Magazine: Deborah Solomon, "The Skinny on Politics: Questions for Mike Huckabee," *New York Times Magazine*, Aug. 7, 2005, p. 14.

189 *In November 2005, the University of Michigan:* "Women's Health: The Press and Public Policy," conference held at the University of Michigan, Nov. 7, 2005.

189 *And there it was, in the pile of yellow slips of paper:* The author was a panelist at the conference.

189 *Then Michigan's surgeon general, Kimberlydawn Wisdom:* Panel discussion at the conference; also, Kimerlydawn Wisdom, interview with the author, Nov. 7, 2005.

189 *The program describes itself as:* Michigan Steps Up, http://www.cacvoices.org/main.asp?a=2&b=0&pageid=655&view=.

190 *"There are economic and professional interests . . .":* Abigail Saguy, interview with the author, Apr. 1, 2005; also, Gina Kolata, "Still Counting on Calorie Counting: Study Aside, Fat-Fighting Industry Vows to Stick to Its Mission," *New York Times*, Apr. 29, 2005, p. C1.

190 *"A lot of the reasons that perceptions about obesity . . .":* Jeffrey Friedman, interview with the author, Mar. 30, 2005.

190 *They've been doing so for years:* Gary D. Foster, interview with the author, July 15, 2004.

190 *(It's a study sponsored by the almond industry . . .):* University of Pennsylvania, http://www.med.upenn.edu/weight/research.shtml.

191 *At Yale, for example, the same building:* Yale University, http://www.yale.edu/ ycewd/.

191 *Its director, Kelly Brownell, who also directs:* Kelly D. Brownell and Katherine Battle Horgen, *Food Fight: The Inside Story of the Food Industry, America's Obesity Crisis, and What We Can Do About It* (New York: McGraw-Hill, 2004), pp. 60–199.

191 *There was, for example, a CDC study that Julie Gerberding:* Author listened to the telephone press conference given by Julie Gerberding on June 2, 2005; also, Gina Kolata, "C.D.C. Investigates Outbreak of Obesity," *New York Times*, June 3, 2005, p. A18.

192 *"We were looking at our data," explained:* Kolata, "C.D.C. Investigates," p. A18.

192 *"My God," he said:* Daniel McGee, interview with the author, June 2, 2005.

193 *On October 3, 2005, the Rand Corporation:* Rand Corporation, http://www .rand.org/news/press.05/10.05.html.

194 *"Everyone has a deeply held set of beliefs . . .":* Jeffrey Friedman, interview with the author, June 1, 2004.

194 *But, notes David Williamson, an obesity researcher:* David Williamson, interview with the author, Dec. 15, 2004.

194 *"It looks like food intake per capita is declining . . .":* Jeffrey Friedman, interview with the author, June 1, 2004.

194 *One problem with looking at national statistics:* Jules Hirsch, interview with the author, Mar. 22, 2004.

194 *"We're different creatures than we used to be," Hirsch says:* Ibid.

195 *"You can't possibly saturate the country . . .":* Ibid.

195 *"If you are on the political right . . .":* Kolata, "Still Counting on Calorie Counting," p. C1.

195 *That was grim, David Satcher, the surgeon general, announced:* Office of the U.S. Surgeon General, http://www.surgeongeneral.gov/news/pressreleases/ pr_obesity.htm.

195 *The surgeon general's report, "A Call to Action . . .":* James Morone, interview with the author, Apr. 5, 2004; also, Kolata, "Still Counting on Calorie Counting," p. C1.

196 *"The operative term," says Sander Gilman, a distinguished professor:* Sander Gilman, interview with the author, May 1, 2005; also, Kolata, "Still Counting on Calorie Counting," p. C1.

196 *"If you can play the child card or the youth card . . .":* Abigail Saguy, interview with the author, Apr. 1, 2005.

196 *The obesity moral panic had a "cultural resonance," Saguy notes:* Abigail Saguy, interview with the author, Apr. 1, 2005; also, Kolata, "Still Counting on Calorie Counting," p. C1.

196 *"Things we didn't think were possible before . . .":* Ibid.

196 *At the same time, Saguy said, the moral panic over obesity:* Abigail Saguy, interview with the author, Apr. 1, 2005.

197 *One was an eight-year, $20 million project:* Benjamin Caballero et al., "Pathways: A School-Based Randomized Controlled Trial for the Prevention of Obesity in American Indian Schoolchildren," *American Journal of Clinical Nutrition,* Nov. 2003, vol. 78, no. 5, pp. 1030–1038.

197 *He explains the study design:* Benjamin Caballero, interview with the author, Nov. 10, 2005.

198 *And here's the indicator that was perhaps most surprising: American Journal of Clinical Nutrition,* http://www.ajcn.org/.

198 *When asked about that:* Benjamin Caballero, e-mail to author, Oct. 10, 2005.

199 *It included 5,106 children from ninety-six schools:* Philip R. Nader et al., "Three-Year Maintenance of Improved Diet and Physical Activity," *Archives of Pediatrics and Adolescent Medicine,* 1999, vol. 163, pp. 695–704.

199 *Even the National Institutes of Health:* National Heart, Lung, and Blood Institute, http://www.nhlbi.nih.gov/health/public/heart/obesity/wecan/.

200 *"There is some social pressure to do something":* Benjamin Caballero, interview with the author, Nov. 11, 2005.

200 *It reminds one scientist, David Freedman:* David Freedman, interview with the author, Feb. 10, 2006.

201 *They began, they say, because they saw:* Katherine Flegal and David Williamson, interviews with and e-mails to the author, 2004 and 2005.

201 *Shortly after they began, one of their colleagues:* David Allison et al., "Annual Deaths Attributable to Obesity in the United States," *Journal of the American Medical Association,* 1999, vol. 282, pp. 1530–1538.

201 *But when Flegal and Williamson read that paper:* Katherine Flegal and David Williamson, interviews with the author, 2004 and 2005.

202 *Finally, it appeared in the* American Journal of Public Health*:* Katherine Flegal et al., "Estimating Deaths Attributable to Obesity in the United States," *American Journal of Public Health,* 2004, vol. 94, pp. 1486–1489.

203 *In the meantime, the* Journal of the American Medical Association*:* Ali H. Mokdad et al., "Actual Causes of Death in the United States, 2000," *Journal of the American Medical Association,* 2004, vol. 291, pp. 1238–1245.

204 *Flegal's paper, written with her colleagues:* Katherine Flegal et al., "Excess Deaths Associated with Underweight, Overweight, and Obesity," *Journal of the American Medical Association,* 2005, vol. 293, pp. 1861–1867.

204 *Barbara Hulka, an emerita professor of epidemiology:* Barbara Hulka, interview with the author, Apr. 18, 2005.

204 *Daniel McGee, the Florida State University statistician:* Daniel McGee, interview with the author, Apr. 18, 2005.

205 *"It's called the obesity paradox," Williamson said:* David Williamson, interview with the author, Apr. 15, 2005.

205 *The new paper, noted Frank Hu, an associate professor:* Frank Hu, Harvard School of Public Health seminar, May 26, 2005. The author watched the streaming video of the seminar.

205 *Scott M. Grundy, a heart researcher:* Scott M. Grundy, ibid.

205 *"That can lead to serious underestimates . . .":* JoAnn Manson, ibid.

205 *Walter Willett, a professor of epidemiology and nutrition:* Walter Willett, interview with the author, May 26, 2005.

205 *None of that was true, Flegal said:* Katherine Flegal, interviews with and e-mails to the author, May 2005.

206 *"We have data sets that are truly nationally representative . . .":* David Williamson, interviews with the author, Apr., May, and Aug. 2005.

206 *"This whole thing is a really strange mix . . .":* Barry Graubard, interview with the author, Sept. 9, 2005.

206 *"I don't know what to say . . .":* Katherine Flegal, interview with the author, May 26, 2005.

207 *"Some went after us individually . . .":* David Williamson, interview with the author, Aug. 17, 2005.

207 *"The past year has seen scientific studies . . .":* Harvard School of Public Health, "Despite Conflicting Studies About Obesity, Most Americans Think the Problem Remains Serious," press release, July 14, 2005. Available from http://www.hsph.harvard.edu/press/releases/press07142005.html.

208 *Writing in the June 2005 issue, he said:* James O. Hill, "Is Obesity Bad?" editorial, *Obesity Management*, June 2005, vol. 1, no. 1, p. 86.

209 *When the researchers drew graphs of heights:* Robert William Fogel, *The Escape from Hunger and Premature Death, 1700–2100: Europe, America, and the Third World* (Cambridge, Eng.: Cambridge University Press, 2004), pp. 23–32.

209 *"We don't know that yet," Fogel says:* Robert W. Fogel, interview with the author, Apr. 5, 2006.

210 *"That's what bothers me," he says:* Barry Graubard, interview with the author, Sept. 9, 2005.

210 *The study, which took place in Sweden:* L. Sjöström et al., "Lifestyle, Diabetes, and Cardiovascular Risk Factors Ten Years After Bariatric Surgery," *New England Journal of Medicine*, Dec. 23, 2004, vol. 351, pp. 2683–2693.

211 *The study, published in the* New England Journal of Medicine *in 2004:* Samuel Klein et al., "Absence of an Effect of Liposuction on Insulin Action and Risk Factors for Coronary Disease," June 17, 2004, vol. 350, pp. 2549–2557.

211 *"Our results suggest . . .":* Ibid., p. 2556.

211 *"If you are obese and don't have comorbidities . . .":* Jeffrey Friedman, interview with the author, Mar. 30, 2005.

EPILOGUE

220 *"If psychology ever taught us anything . . .":* Peter Herman, interview with the author, Aug. 5, 2004.

222 *He said that this was the typical response:* Gina Kolata, *Ultimate Fitness: The Quest for Truth About Exercise and Health* (New York: Farrar, Straus and Giroux, 2003), p. 46.

Acknowledgments

I am deeply indebted to all of the scientists and dieters who are quoted and cited in this book. But I owe a special debt to the stalwart dieters in the Penn group who graciously allowed me to sit in on their meetings and, especially, to Carmen Pirollo, Graziella Mann, Jerry Gordon, and Ron Krauss, who spoke to me at length and told me their stories.

Several scientists in particular were extremely helpful and I am appreciative of their efforts. Jeff Friedman, Rudy Leibel, Jules Hirsch, Mickey Stunkard, and Stephen O'Rahilly patiently answered question after question and helped me enormously in my efforts to be accurate and fair. Katherine Flegal and David Williamson supplied statistics and tutorials on the interpretation of data. Gary Foster provided my entrée to the Penn group and gave me candid and informative assessments of diet research.

I also am grateful to Paul Elie, my editor at Farrar, Straus and Giroux, whose insights shaped this book.

And, as always, I am thankful to my husband, Bill, who read draft after draft of my manuscript and unstintingly gave me his honest comments.

Index